HEALTH
The Foundations for
Achievement

This edition is dedicated to the memory of my mother and father, who would not have been in the least surprised by all the fuss the first edition caused.

HEALTH
The Foundations for Achievement

SECOND EDITION

David Seedhouse
*Auckland University of Technology, New Zealand
and Middlesex University, London, UK*

JOHN WILEY & SONS, LTD
Chichester · New York · Weinheim · Brisbane · Singapore · Toronto

Other Wiley Editorial Offices

John Wiley & Sons Inc., 111 River Street, Hoboken, NJ 07030, USA

Jossey-Bass, 989 Market Street, San Francisco, CA 94103-1741, USA

Wiley-VCH Verlag GmbH, Boschstr. 12, D-69469 Weinheim, Germany

John Wiley & Sons Australia Ltd, 33 Park Road, Milton, Queensland 4064, Australia

John Wiley & Sons (Asia) Pte Ltd, 2 Clementi Loop #02-01, Jin Xing Distripark, Singapore 129809

John Wiley & Sons Canada Ltd, 22 Worcester Road, Etobicoke, Ontario, Canada M9W 1L1

Wiley also publishes its books in a variety of electronic formats. Some content that
appears in print may not be available in electronic books.

Library of Congress Cataloging-in-Publication Data

Seedhouse, David
  Health : the foundations for achievment / David Seedhouse. - 2nd ed.
     p. cm.
  Includes bibliographical references and index.
  ISBN 0-471-49011-3
  1. Health. I. Title.

  RA776.S445 2001
  613 - dc21   2001024350

British Library Cataloguing in Publication Data

A catalogue record for this book is available from the British Library

ISBN 10: 0-471-49011-3
ISBN 13: 978-0-471-49011-1

Typeset in 10/12 pt Palatino from the author's disks by Dobbie Typesetting Limited, Tavistock, Devon

This book is printed on acid-free paper responsibly manufactured from sustainable forestry
in which at least two trees are planted for each one used for paper production.

Contents

Foreword   vii

Preface   ix

Preface to the First Edition   xi

Acknowledgements   xv

Introduction to the Second Edition   1

Chapter One   What is Health?   5

Chapter Two   The Need for Philosophy   15

Chapter Three   The Problem of Meaning   23

Chapter Four   Theories of Health   37

Chapter Five   The Fullest Sense of Health   81

Chapter Six   The Idea of Human Potential   103

Chapter Seven   The Assessment of the Health of Individuals   109

Chapter Eight   The Aims of Health Education and Promotion   121

Chapter Nine   How Can Health for All be Achieved?   133

References   135

Index   139

Foreword

I am honoured to have been asked to write a foreword for *Health: The Foundations for Achievement*. When I was teaching nurse practitioners in the early nineties, I recommended the first edition as a course book. I thought it was quite radical in the way it dealt with health. I was also working at that time as a nurse practitioner in a shelter for single homeless men, and that reminded me constantly about my own and others' assumptions about what health is. Most medical visitors to the hostel spent a long time talking to the men about stopping smoking. The men clearly thought these visitors were crazy: imagine worrying about smoking when your 'home' is the size of a single bed and a locker, with all the privacy and amenities you might expect. At that time, I welcomed being able to think about health as a foundation for achievement – where I could have a legitimate concern with basic needs of food and drink, shelter, warmth and a purpose in life as foundations for health, and still be a nurse practitioner!

The publication of this second edition finds me in a markedly different set of circumstances. Now I work for the World Health Organization. I wondered would the volume have the same relevance for me, as I struggle with concepts of 'health' in developing countries. Things didn't look too promising at first: the book takes a strong stance against the tensions between what WHO stands for (the ideal state of health) and what it does (concerns itself with disease). I wondered if I had somehow sold out!

I work in some of the world's poorest countries, collaborating with staff there to develop strong health systems. *Their* major concerns, and so mine, are low life expectancy, the devastation of HIV/AIDS, preventable maternal and child deaths and the overwhelming burden of disease. Little wonder, looking at this short list, that it is tempting to run for the cover of medical interventions and cure or prevention: WHO and its staff become disease focused, despite the heady ideals of health as perfect well being (see Chapter 4 for a full discussion of this issue). But of course other factors have a strong influence on health – poverty, war, literacy and hunger. And David Seedhouse is right – it is easier to acknowledge the breadth of factors which impact on health, than it is to design interventions to address them. So apparently we end up with some dissonance.

The challenge for all of us in health care, whether in WHO, in developing countries or in a local general practice, is learning to live with things that don't fit – with the dissonance of the way the world works. My work in systems development reminds me all the time that relationships are not linear in systems, and there is little which is not part of a system. To take one example, the WHO programme on TB is, of course, concerned with the diagnosis and treatment of TB. But if you were to look closely, you would see that it has a strong programme on community development, because that's where TB happens, and that's where the solutions to TB must start. Their programme on community development is concerned with housing, economics, education, volunteers – anything, in fact, which concerns communities. But it doesn't altogether 'fit' in what a programme entitled 'Tuberculosis' might be expected to contain. And community development might not fit into a country's programme. Why not? Well, an impoverished country might find it easier to get a donor to develop a TB programme than to develop a programme in community health. Or TB might be such a problem in that country that other developments must address what for them is a priority. Community development might offer a 'vehicle' to all kinds of other developments, but it is not the country priority, no matter what I, as a health systems adviser, privy to the big picture, might say.

And when you think about this, it is not so different from considering the context and meaning of health for any individual, family or group. They will have their priorities too – built around their pressing needs, culture, current concerns and social structures. What I (as a health professional) identify as their most urgent needs may not be the barrier to health which they identify. They, like countries, are the owners of their own big picture – the needs which for them represent real barriers to health. Their solutions must fit into their big picture as well as mine.

The strength of this volume for me, now, is that it is a helpful companion with which to explore this business of 'fit' in health. It steers me down a road which says that it's OK not to know the answers, as long as I don't lose the wide focus of my view, and consider and reconsider the barriers to achievement of health.

One of the teachings of Buddha begins: 'We do not need more knowledge but more wisdom', and as I have been reading the second edition I have been repeatedly reminded of these words. I suppose it's a function of age, but I seem to spend a lot of time these days looking back at changed views – what seemed so clear, obvious and right to me twenty years ago now seems less of a certainty. My steadily accruing knowledge does not seem to lead to a sense of being equipped with all the answers. It has been reassuring to share David Seedhouse's reflective journey through his thoughts in this second edition of this book. This is not a journey in which he tells us how wrong he was in 1985, but one in which he openly reflects on how his thinking about health has developed over those intervening years. Whether you are a new practitioner or an experienced one, sure of yourself or full of uncertainty, I urge you to enjoy this opportunity for reflection and discussion about health.

Barbara Stilwell
Department of Organization of Health Services Delivery
WHO, Geneva
April 2001

Preface

Much has changed in the fifteen years since I wrote the first edition of this book, and yet nothing has changed. I have moved on. I know more about the conventional health world than I did. My thinking has developed. And yet basically the whole of my philosophy of health is here – based on the apparently obvious insight that work for health is work to remove any obstacle to fulfilling human potential, and not just the obstacles of disease and illness.

The conventional health world has moved on too. Courses on communication and ethics for health professionals are now commonplace (they were rare in 1985). Fifteen years ago mention of the philosophy of health produced puzzlement at best and ridicule at worst, but it is now respectable – there are even one or two university posts in the subject. And yet nothing has really changed. Health is popularly associated solely with clinical matters, the medical profession is as powerful an influence as ever, bioethics has become a specialism in its own right – so perpetuating the idea that health (even where ethics is concerned) is the province of experts, and health promoters around the world say they are promoting health holistically while they concern themselves almost entirely with disease prevention.

But then change takes time. Re-writing this book has convinced me that the **foundations theory of health** is theoretically coherent and robust, and also practically applicable. Furthermore, it is surely the most extensive theory of its kind in existence, and yet it still has great potential for further improvement. It has spawned several subsequent books, and many other ideas and practical decision-making devices (all of which – including the Ethical Grid – are based on the reasoning first advanced in this book).

I have also been reminded that perhaps the time for the philosophy of health has not yet come. I can imagine, a few years from now (given good work by committed practical philosophers and health workers), that the philosophy of health could have an equivalent status and influence to the philosophy of science – but maybe not yet. I suspect that at the moment most readers use *Foundations* for its readability and its exposition of competing theories of health – and both these aspects remain, I hope in improved form. Nevertheless, I urge readers old and new to examine the rest of the book more closely – and in particular to try to understand the logic behind the **foundations theory**, and to reflect on its practical application (both tasks ought to be easier in this new edition).

Note finally that I have moved on too far to re-edit the book altogether. To have done so I would have had to write a different book. Consequently, I have kept the character of the original as far as possible – deliberately preserving some ambiguities. As best I can I have reduced repetition (though I have not entirely eliminated it), improved clarity, and tried to achieve a slightly smoother style. I have added extra material within the book, and have also appended an update at the foot of each chapter (except **Chapter Nine**). The updates are – I hope – especially clarifying, and also elucidate the ambiguities retained from the original.

I look back on this book fondly, almost like a father views the work of his son, and yet I haven't changed so much either. I still have – in my work at least – a necessary naïvety. I write about huge issues – the nature of ethics, the goals of health work, the purpose of health policy – while the world 'solves' them, generally irrationally and unfairly, certainly unsystematically. And just as much as ever, I realise that the only way to continue to do what I do is to believe that clear thinking has a part to play in changing the world for the better.

David Seedhouse
Auckland, New Zealand

Preface to the First Edition

This book poses two fundamental questions. These are: 'what is health?' and 'how can more health be achieved?' There have been several previous attempts to answer these questions. They form part of a continuing debate which has confusion and ambiguity as its main characteristic. This book, by viewing the debate from a novel perspective, clears away misunderstanding, clarifies the basic issues, and probes the surprising consequences of this clarification.

The book is a gauntlet thrown at the feet of people who claim to be working for health. Although in practice much excellent caring work is done despite this confusion, many 'health workers' have set their sights too low. Disease and illness pose real obstacles to be overcome, but preventing and curing disease and illness is not the whole story of work for health. By working to change only such factors as poor diet and smoking habits, or by prescribing drugs intended to alleviate symptoms brought about by the wider pressures of life, 'health workers' are digging only shallow foundations.

What has emerged from the volumes of writing on health is an indigestible spaghetti of confusion. The word 'health' is already defined in dictionaries, and used everyday as if it is fully understood. In Britain there is a National Health Service and a Minister of Health, there are Health Centres, Health Farms, and academic departments of Health Studies. Health Visitors practise in the community and there are expanding groups working for Health Education and Health Promotion, staffed by professionally qualified Health Education and Health Promotion Officers who devote their careers to increasing health. Consequently it might seem a little late to be asking 'what is health?' Surely it must be true that people who are working for health know, by definition, what health is.

In spite of all this the fact remains that it is not clear what is being talked about when health is discussed. The word 'health' is used to mean many different things. For a medic health might mean physical fitness, absence of disease, or the harmonious functioning of the organs of the body. For an administrator in a hospital health might mean the state of a person when that person is discharged; for a member of the World Health Organisation health might mean complete physical, social and mental well-being; for a health educator health might be essentially a freedom to make choices about personal habits and activities, and for a social scientist health might mean a person's ability to function according to social customs and norms – or it might mean the opposite of this if the scientist does not think these norms desirable. Much depends upon the particular profession or interest of whoever is seeking health. Different professions work with different theories of health, and in turn these theories may not be the same as those of the lay people they are trying to serve.

Does a person's health depend on where he lives? Does a person's health depend upon the sort of society in which she lives? Does health vary according to a person's gender? Or according to a person's race? Or according to a person's age? Do doctors work for full health? Is the National Health Service a misnomer? It is possible to study for a Diploma of Health Education at some British Polytechnics, but even on these courses it is not made fully clear what health education actually is, or should be.

These and many other questions need to be tackled urgently, and the web of confusion that has been fostered by ambiguity must be untangled. The extent of the ambiguity can be disconcerting. People expect to be able to specify the nature of health. If the symptoms of illnesses and diseases can be described fairly precisely it is natural to think that health too ought to be describable in a fairly precise way. However, it is not so easy; issues about the nature of health are complicated and contentious. 'Health' is one of a number of words which are constantly in use which are so rich in meaning that they cannot be explained fully without invoking controversy. This poses a challenge for us to try to understand more clearly what we mean when we use such words, and to pinpoint limits beyond which we do not wish to use them. To understand the problems involved and to arrive at a proper view of the full sense of health requires effort. It is not possible, even if it were desirable, to lead a student of health by the hand to an indisputable conclusion. The student must work to see the point of alternative theories, to recognise the difficulties involved with each, and then to arrive at a considered opinion.

The primary aim of this book is to clarify the meanings and sense of the word 'health'. It is naturally appealing to try to change the human condition by a frontal attack, to try to cure injustice, poverty, sickness, drabness, and the inhuman treatment of people by their fellow men with urgent action, but the track record of previous such interventions is not good. Cautious preparation is essential. It is far better first to clarify the ground from which to work, to know that what is to be said has been thoroughly thought through, and that the position can be properly defended against attack. This is the reason for doing philosophy. This is a central aim of this book.

Because of this need for a careful preparation some patience is required to read the book. At times the discussion is almost purely theoretical. Such puzzling about abstract issues may irritate practitioners who are used to trying to solve urgent problems by direct action. Even though the approach of the book is at all times appropriate to real problems of life one objection will inevitably be raised. This is one version of it:

> We know what is wrong with society and the British health service already. Why bother with the preliminaries? Why write this sort of book at all?
>
> What is the point of writing a book that tries first and foremost to get to the roots of meaning and sense of a single word? Surely there are many more relevant directions along which to press an inquiry than to pursue abstract clarification and discussion of ideas. Our world is beset by real problems which are clear enough already. Within and between societies there are gross inequalities of wealth, power, quality of life, opportunity, food and housing resources. Enormous sums of money are spent on military research and on arming some nations with a thousand-times more destructive power than is needed to

annihilate the entire Earth, while at the same time people are dying of starvation. Only a privileged few are able to develop themselves intellectually by attending centres of higher education, while others go through life only barely literate and numerate, either to work long hours for low pay – or not to work at all; and our world is suffering from the pollution of land, sea, and air as a result of short-sighted industrial policies and processes.

There are so many blatant wrongs to be righted that scepticism about the worth of an investigation into a word – six black letters on a white page – seems fully justified. Such scepticism might be appropriate if the pursuit of health were to be abandoned following clarification, but the clarifying process is only one part of the project. Because of the work done to clear the ground properly it becomes possible to put forward a more precise and comprehensive theory of health than has ever been offered before.

Health should be thought of as the *foundations for achievement*. Health is not a single goal which can be universally achieved – health has degrees and levels just as different sorts of buildings have different sorts and standards of foundations. These foundations are not merely those required for biological or physical achievement. They are those required for a wide range of human achievement, including the biological but also encompassing emotional, intellectual, spiritual, creative, and recreational potentials. Some of the foundations which make up a person's health are essential to enable any human being to achieve anything worthwhile.

The implications of this new theory of health are huge. To win the battle for fuller health there must be major changes in the education system, in freedom of access to information, and in the system of basic welfare in societies. Health is already a significant political issue, but the issue is far more explosive than many who advocate the dismantling or the expansion of the health service, or existing systems of 'health care' in other societies, realise.

David Seedhouse
Stockport, England
September 1985

Acknowledgements

I would like to thank my friends, Alan Cribb and Harry Lesser, all the members of the Oldham WEA philosophy group who endured my ramblings and misconceptions about health, Dr Michael Wilson and Dr Rosemary Biggs. All challenged my ideas and pointed out better directions to take.

I would also like to thank all the friends, colleagues and students who – over the last fifteen years – have boosted my sometimes flagging confidence that this research project is worth doing.

I am grateful for permission to use copyright material:

Arthur Koestler (1969), *The Act of Creation*, Hutchinson, London, pp. 118–120. Printed by permission of A. D. Peters & Co. Ltd.

Alexander Solzhenitsyn, *Cancer Ward*, pp. 467–468. English translation ©1969 by The Bodley Head. Reprinted by permission of Farrar, Straus & Giroux, Inc., New York.

Introduction to the Second Edition

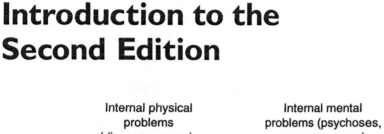

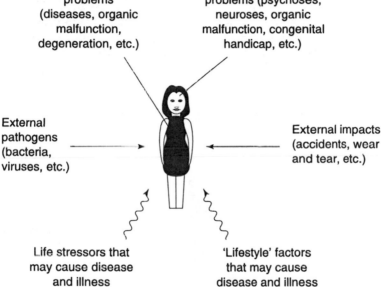

Internal physical problems (diseases, organic malfunction, degeneration, etc.)

Internal mental problems (psychoses, neuroses, organic malfunction, congenital handicap, etc.)

External pathogens (bacteria, viruses, etc.)

External impacts (accidents, wear and tear, etc.)

Life stressors that may cause disease and illness

'Lifestyle' factors that may cause disease and illness

AN INDIVIDUAL WITH A HEALTH PROBLEM

Figure I   The conventional conception of health

Generally speaking, there are three different ways to conceive of health. **Figure 1** is the **first conception**.

This is the contemporary medical understanding of health, according to which health problems exist in individuals. On this conception, it is believed that in most or even all cases health problems should be dealt with by applying clinical techniques to specific parts of individual bodies or minds.

Medicine is interested in how these problems are caused, but only secondarily. What matters most is dealing with health problems as the clinical system encounters them.

This **image of health** currently overwhelms the thinking of governments, policy-makers and news media throughout the Western world, and our 'health systems' – and therefore a sizeable proportion of our life experience and expectations – are shaped by it.

It is, however, quite impossible to prove that this is the correct or objective conception of health, and there are alternative understandings of at least equal plausibility.

Figure 2 is the **second conception of health**.

This is the socially aware response to the conventional conception. The figure in the diagram is usually considered to be an individual, and disease, illness and injury remain the only sorts of health problems possible. However, on this understanding the figure may also be thought of as a collection of people – a family, a community, a vulnerable group, an underprivileged social stratum – and the causes of health problems are considered at least as important as their cures. Furthermore, cures for health problems are held to lie both within and outside conventional health services.

The conviction behind this conception of health is that a significant proportion of health problems (i.e. problems of disease and illness) are caused by and are therefore **dependent on** environmental and social circumstances (hence the strong arrows in **Figure 2** emanating from 'social and environmental circumstances'). This means that

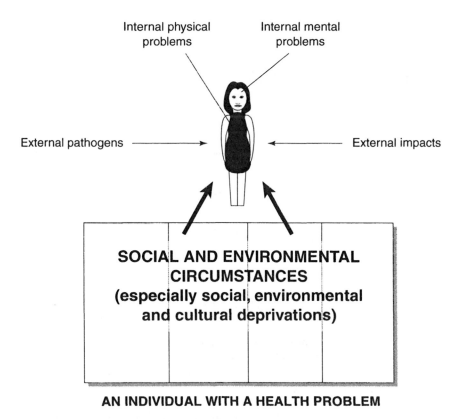

AN INDIVIDUAL WITH A HEALTH PROBLEM

Figure 2   The socially aware conception of health

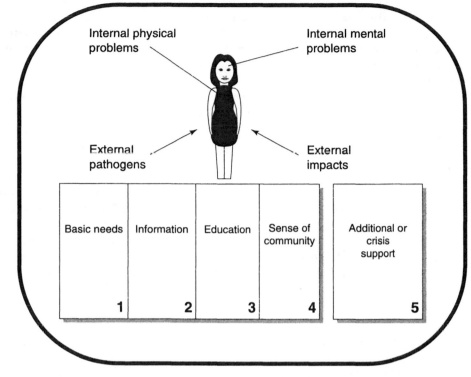

THE STATE OF HEALTH OF AN INDIVIDUAL OR A GROUP

Figure 3   The foundations conception of health

work for health should concentrate both on providing for people when we are sick and on ensuring that social conditions are improved in order that the incidence of sickness may be reduced. Furthermore, this understanding tends to foster the view that health inequalities – meaning inequalities in morbidity and mortality – between differently privileged people should be reduced, and ideally made equal.

There is also a **third conception of health**, which looks like **Figure 3**.

This is a holistic understanding of health which recognises both that health problems can be caused by agents of disease, and that problems of disease and illness often have social and environmental causes. However, the **foundations understanding of health** does not accept that there is a special distinction between problems of disease and illness and other problems of life. The theory embraces the logical implication of this and consequently extends its conception of health as follows:

a. **Health problems are not only problems of health and disease**, rather they are problems of autonomy (of moving on our foundations for achievement). Roughly speaking, the more autonomy we have the greater our health: the better our foundations for achievement the more health we enjoy.

b. The foundations figure's state of health is **not only dependent on the platform, it is equivalent to the state of the conditions which provide for autonomous movement** on the foundations stage. **Everything within the circle in Figure 3 must be considered in any assessment of the foundations figure's state of health**. There are no arrows emanating from the stage because some or all of a person's or a group's health simply *is* the stage.

c. **Health work – and therefore health services – based on the foundations image should aim as a priority to reinforce the foundations figure's platform for achievement**. They should include medical services in so far as these support the foundations figure's autonomy, but this specialised branch of human endeavour should not dictate health policy.

The **first conception** thinks of the foundations figure as largely or entirely **separate from** social and environmental influences (and those wedded to it certainly tend to act as if this is so when they administer therapy[1,2]). The **second conception** recognises the role of social and environmental factors in **causing** health problems (i.e. problems of disease and illness). The **third conception** sees social, environmental and personal factors as **part of** the foundations figure's state of health – and therefore proposes a radical re-focusing of health work. On this image disease and illness are no longer central to work for health – what matters fundamentally is what we are able to do with our lives.

I did not intend to make these distinctions when I set out to write the first edition of this book. I wanted merely to understand the nature of health. However, the logic is irresistible – if all theories of and approaches to health are directed against obstacles to fulfilling human potential then there cannot possibly be a demarcation between problems of disease and other problems. Once this is accepted everything in health care looks different.

This book (in its first edition) was the initial step in an exploration of just how different health care might become. Readers familiar with my subsequent work will recognise anticipations of arguments and decision-making tools contained in later texts. Indeed it should be obvious that all the ensuing work depends on this book's analysis. However, the book should be enjoyed most for what it was at the time it was written: an enthusiastic, optimistic, socially concerned (and – to me at least – endearingly naïve) philosophical foray into a question largely disregarded by philosophers.

CHAPTER ONE

What is Health?

THE CHALLENGE

The challenge is to discover what health means and to explain how more of it can be achieved.

The word 'health' is used in many different ways. People often say they 'have health', 'are healthy' or live in a 'healthy society'. We claim 'healthy appetites' and 'healthy attitudes'. We may be 'health educators', eat 'health food' or work in faculties of 'health studies'. And we sometimes declare we are healthy just because we live in democracies, families, or happily on our own.

Scholars and practitioners continue to debate the meaning of health. Some hold that the correct definition is that *health is a commodity*, others consider *health an ideal state*, others believe an individual is healthy so long as she is *able to function normally*, and yet others claim that *health is a reserve of strength* which helps us adapt to changing circumstances.

Which uses are correct? Which are important? And which are trivial? Is there a common theme that links them all? Where they conflict, how can we decide which to accept and which to reject?

It is the purpose of this book to answer these questions.

Two points must be made clear at the outset:

1. To discover the meaning of health it is not enough to consult a dictionary

Dictionaries are not oracles, and those who compile them do not have sovereignty over the meanings of words. Dictionaries are written by particular people with particular values who live in particular societies and eras. It is perfectly possible to disagree with dictionary definitions and to have good reasons for doing so.

Raymond Williams – a 20th century writer and academic – pointedly demonstrated the folly of placing oneself in servitude to someone else's view of the world. He commented that:

> Some people, when they see a word, think the first thing to do is define it. Dictionaries are produced and, with a show of authority no less confident because it is so limited in place

and time, what is called a proper meaning is attached. I once began collecting, from correspondence in newspapers, and from other public arguments, variations on the phrases 'I see from my Webster' and 'I find from my Oxford dictionary'. Usually what was at issue was a difficult term in an argument. But the effective tone of these phrases, with their interesting overture of possession ('my Webster'), was to appropriate a meaning which fitted the argument and to exclude those meanings which were inconvenient to it but which some benighted person had been so foolish as to use. Of course if we want to be clear about...barber, or barley, or barn, this kind of definition is effective. But for words of a different kind, and especially for those which involve ideas and values, it is not only an impossible but an irrelevant procedure. (Williams, 1976, pp. 14–15)[3]

The idea of health is not to be found within the pages of a dictionary. The nature of health is disputed and different understandings can be legitimately held. No matter how established the source, no one has privileged access to health's true meaning.

2.   It is not enough to say that health is desirable and bad health undesirable

It seems obvious that health is desirable and bad health not, and yet no human desire is universally held. It is not even true that all human beings desire to be free from disease and illness:

i.   Some diseases are culturally defined, which means that what is regarded as a disease in one culture may be regarded as normal – or even desirable – in another. Lester King gives the example of foot-binding in China, a practice which caused women considerable pain and disability as they sought or were forced to be fashionable (or to conform to social norms).[4] Women's feet were tightly bound from childhood – producing what present-day Westerners would call serious disfigurement and restricted mobility – yet the women were not considered diseased, ill or disabled.

According to present day Western social norms, these women would be considered injured at least.

ii.   It is well known that disease and illness is sometimes desired – even courted – in order to avoid work, engender sympathy, or obtain privilege.

iii.   Some people are prepared to accept disease in order to achieve higher goals. Long-term disaster relief workers, for example, expect to contract illness as a part of their work. Though they would presumably rather not become ill, they nevertheless place themselves in situations where they risk sickness they could easily have avoided by staying home.

As soon as one asks serious questions about *what health is* it becomes obvious that it is not enough to respond 'health is desirable' since this is as uninformative as answering the question 'what is happiness?' with 'everyone wants it'. Such a reply tells us nothing about the subject in question.

Generalisation seems to lead to a blind alley. Instead, let us briefly examine the question 'what is health?' at the level of everyday life, by contemplating real people in real situations.

WHEN IS A PERSON HEALTHY?

If it is possible to say that some people are healthy and others not this should provide important clues about the meaning of health.

THE CASE STUDIES

The following studies are presented both to further this inquiry into the meaning of health and to provoke thought in the reader.

After each case the reader should ask:

1. **Is the person healthy?**

2. **If he is, why? If not, why is he unhealthy?**

3. **How might she be made healthier?**

CASE ONE

PERCY

Percy is a 36 year-old white bachelor who has worked as a clerk for various firms. In his last post he was responsible for the sale and despatch of spare parts for cranes. Six years ago, during an economic recession, he was made redundant by the crane company. Since then he has had to make do with various kinds of temporary work, usually manual, and has drawn unemployment benefit when nothing else was available.

Three years ago Percy began to suffer from occasional delusions over which he had no control. He would believe he was another person, taking on that person's character and acting exactly as if he were that person. Sometimes the people he imagined himself to be were real and known to him, at other times they were invented. The delusions never lasted longer than three hours, and afterwards Percy could remember nothing about what had happened.

Once Percy acted as if he was the office manager at the crane company. One lunchtime he took over a desk at the office of the builder for whom he was working as a temporary labourer and managed to order eight jib sections of cranes which were then invoiced to the building firm. On another occasion he imagined he was Bruce Springsteen − a hero of long-standing − and ran up an overdraft of $5000 in one day at various clothing and musical instrument shops.

Recently Percy has sought professional help. He knows he cannot expect to hold down a job if his present problem continues, since his sporadic delusions make it impossible for people to treat him normally. At the time of each hallucination no one can communicate

continues

— *continued* —

with Percy. They have to interact with Bruce, or whoever else he is at the time. Percy consulted his GP who referred him to a psychiatrist. Both doctors could find nothing physically wrong with Percy and could not pin down a mental illness.

Perhaps surprisingly Percy has no disease which medical science can label with certainty, though it has been suggested he might become a voluntary patient at the local hospital for mental illness and be assessed further.

CASE TWO

DENNIS

Dennis is a 45-year-old white man. He has worked as a bank teller for twenty years, and has been at his present branch for the last eight of these. He is rather flabby but not over-weight according to the norm for his height and body structure. He is married and lives in England in a smallish three-bedroomed semi-detached house on an estate built just before the Second World War. He has no children.

Dennis returns home from work each day and can do no more than eat his evening meal – which is always prepared by his wife – and then doze in front of the television before retiring to bed. At weekends Dennis likes to 'lie-in' until at least midday. He enjoys watching TV sports programmes and spends the bulk of his spare time idly viewing the various subscriber channels.

Out of habit, Dennis visits his local GP once a year for a check-up. As far as anyone knows Dennis has no diseases, and he does not feel ill.

CASE THREE

ANNE

Anne is a white woman of 32. She suffered a serious car accident whilst working as a journalist for a popular women's magazine. A vehicle overtaking from the opposite direction forced her off the road, causing her to collide at speed with an irresistible brick wall. She had greatly enjoyed her work, which involved writing special features and travelling to report from the scene of dramatic news events.

Unfortunately, as a result of the accident she is now a paraplegic – her lower limbs and most of her torso are paralysed. She lives in a specially designed flat, on her own since her

continues

continued

husband left because 'she is not the woman she was'. And yet today she is content, caring, and always tries to encourage others, whatever their problem. She receives help from health and social service workers, provided by the state from tax revenue.

Anne has a good income from the interest from compensation received from the insurers of the driver of the car that precipitated the crash, and from payment for regular articles for various magazines on a freelance basis. She now specialises in writing for periodicals for disabled people.

CASE FOUR

BETTY

Betty is a white, 'middle-class' widow aged 51. She has three children, two of whom are married and have left home. She lives, in a house she owns outright, with her 16-year-old youngest son. He is taking pre-university qualifications at his local technical college.

Betty has cancer. Two years ago she had a mastectomy followed by a course of radiation therapy, and then by chemotherapy. She has been feeling 'sick and giddy' recently and has been told that cancer has reappeared as a small but inoperable tumour on her brain. Once again she is having radiation therapy, which is again to be followed by a course of chemotherapy. In addition to her headaches and increasing immobility she knows she will feel intermittent nausea and that her hair will fall out again.

Betty is miserable and very frightened, as much about what will become of her young son – who is now stealing, lying, and not doing any academic work – than about what will happen to her. However, despite all this she is showing great character and has resolved to fight her disease with all the strength she has. She is determined to survive, at least until she has seen her son move successfully into adult life – something she knows may take several years.

CASE FIVE

THE JAMES FAMILY

Mr and Mrs James are both white and aged 20. They are renting a thirteenth-floor state-owned flat. The wallpaper is peeling from the walls of every room, particularly in the main

continues

continued

bedroom which is noticeably damp. Their electricity supply has recently been cut off because of non-payment of substantial arrears.

Mrs James had an abortion nine months ago. Six weeks ago she took an overdose of Valium and was briefly hospitalised. Last week she discovered she was pregnant again.

When she was a very small child she spent nine weeks 'in care', after which she was brought up by her stepmother. Mother and stepdaughter fell out three years ago and no longer have any contact with each other. Mrs James feels very depressed. She regularly says she cannot go on any more – as far as she can see her life can only get worse.

Mr James is currently on probation for car theft and house-breaking. He has never had paid employment in his life and, although he has tried, has been unable to get a job. The couple's only child is three-and-a-half years old. His speech is slow and he has recurrent bronchitis. He also has frequent temper tantrums.

CASE SIX

WINSTON

Winston is a 22-year-old Maori. All his life he has lived in a small, draughty, cheaply built weather-board house in South Auckland, right next to a busy motorway intersection. He is part of a local gang and is peripherally involved in Maori activism – protesting against colonisation and lack of opportunity for Maori youth.

In common with almost all his friends Winston has never had a full-time job. He deals in 'soft drugs' in a small way in order to supplement his benefit. So far this has been over-looked by the police although Winston is sure they know what he is doing.

Winston has a fine physique and is in excellent shape because he works out every day at the local leisure centre.

CASE SEVEN

PETER

Peter is a 53-year-old American man. He lives in the North-West and is married with two daughters, both of whom are studying at university. He is the CEO of a company trading in cut-glass for the upper range of the market. He lives in a luxurious detached house, which stands in an acre of grounds maintained by a gardener whom Peter employs two

continues

continued

days per week. He has a good circle of friends and acquaintances, enjoys golf, and is active in the local branch of the Republican Party.

Peter lives the 'good life' to the full. He smokes 30 good quality cigarettes a day, often supplemented with two or three cigars. He eats most things heartily but does try to keep his weight down since he cares about his appearance. He drinks three or four bottles of beer — always from local 'boutique breweries' — per day, as well as several single-malt whisky 'chasers'.

Peter is still very ambitious and becomes frustrated easily. Occasionally this frustration becomes manifest in a fit of temper, and twice in the past year he has struck his wife in the face with the palm of his hand.

WHICH OF THESE PEOPLE ARE HEALTHY AND WHICH ARE UNHEALTHY?

In order to reach conclusions about these people's state of health we need to have some idea about what health is, but no clear understanding of health springs from the descriptions of their lives.

This leaves two options. One is to apply existing definitions of health to see how they help answer the question. The other is to attempt a personal assessment of the case studies – to use an intuitive understanding of health – and then work back from this to an explicit account.

1. To take **the first option**, consider the answers one might expect from four hypothetical people, each of whom espouses a different definition of health. They are a *medic*, a *social scientist*, an *idealist* from the World Health Organisation, and a *humanist*.

This particular medic defines health as *the absence of disease, illness and injury*. The social scientist defines health as *the ability to function in a normal social role*. The idealist defines health as *a state of complete physical, mental and social well-being*. And the humanist thinks health is *an ability to adapt positively to the problems of life*.

The Medic

According to the medic *Percy is unhealthy* because he is ill. Although she cannot definitively put a name to Percy's illness she believes the problem is a psychosis of some kind and that further investigation would confirm the type. Certainly, Percy is not clinically normal.

Dennis is healthy, although he does seem to be excessively idle.

Anne is unhealthy - it makes no sense to describe a cripple as healthy. *Betty is unhealthy* because she has cancer. *Mrs James is unhealthy* since she is so depressed. *Mr James is healthy*. The *James child is unhealthy. Winston is very healthy* - he is exceptionally and admirably fit. *Peter is healthy*, but he should watch his smoking and drinking.

The Social Scientist

The problem for the social scientist is to define what a normal social role is. According to this particular scientist it is what a person has been doing for the last three years in which she had no serious disease, illness or injury unusual to her. Consequently, the social scientist thinks *Percy is unhealthy* because he is not functioning in his normal social role. *Dennis is healthy. Anne has regained her health. Betty is unhealthy* because she is unable to do what she used to. *The James family are healthy* - they have had their social roles for over three years. *Winston is healthy* because he has an established way of life. *Peter is healthy* because he has an important social role.

The Idealist

As far as the idealist is concerned *they are all unhealthy*.

The Humanist

The humanist has his own ideas about what positive adaptation is. In his opinion *Percy is healthy* since he is doing what he can to cure himself of his delusions. *Dennis is unhealthy* because he is drifting and doing nothing positive to change his unfulfilling life. *Anne is healthy* because she has adapted excellently to her considerable disabilities. *Betty is healthy* because she is responding positively to her disease and her circumstances. *The James family is unhealthy. Winston is healthy* because he is doing all the positive things he knows, although in the humanist's opinion he could be a lot healthier still if he channelled his energies in other directions. Finally, he thinks *Peter is unhealthy* because the humanist does not consider wife-beating a positive adaptation to stress.

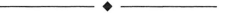

All this is messy and perplexing. Percy, Betty, Mrs James and the James child have been described as unhealthy three times, and as healthy once. Dennis, Anne, Mr James and Peter have each been labelled healthy twice and unhealthy twice. Winston has been described as healthy three times and as unhealthy once.

Undoubtedly, health means different things to different people and it is not easy to see a way to decide between the different understandings.

2.   The **second option** – to attempt a personal assessment of the lives described, without having a definition beforehand – almost inevitably results in puzzlement.

Health issues do not seem to boil down to questions of either/or, so it is very difficult to state definitively that anyone is or isn't healthy. Experience shows that most people want to conclude that the case studies – and indeed all people in real life – are *healthy in some respects even though they are unhealthy in others.* Anne, for example, does not seem to have physical health but she has excellent mental and emotional health. Winston has marvellous physical health but seems badly unfulfilled intellectually and emotionally. Betty is not healthy physically because she has secondary cancer, but she is showing so much resolve, mental strength, stamina, and courage that it is hard to deny that she has a high standard of mental well-being.

This way of looking at the case studies seems to be more balanced, yet it does not advance the inquiry far because it nevertheless allows that *a person can be healthy and unhealthy at the same time.* This seems to be a clear contradiction, on a par with the statement that a person can both be diseased and not diseased at the same time. Later it will become clear that this is not the case; however, we are attempting to answer the question 'what is health?' too early in the investigation. We are not properly prepared, and we do not have a specific theory to test. In order to get to the bottom of the issue – in order to defeat the frustration of not being able to answer a superficially very simple question – it is important to step back from it. It is necessary to see the importance of clarification, to appreciate the extent of the *problem of meaning*, and to recognise the merits and disadvantages of existing theories of health.

WHAT IS HEALTH? – UPDATE

This deceptively simple chapter sets out the challenge for everyone seriously interested in working for health. We talk freely of health. Many of our most important social institutions bear health's name. We imagine we know perfectly well what health means. Yet analysis swiftly undermines our confidence.

First, it is no good saying we all desire health, for this tells us nothing, and in any case we do not always desire the same things. Second, there are several different definitions of health, and once these are applied to real cases it is obvious they are not only dissimilar but incompatible. Third, we cannot rely on unexamined intuitions since they tend to lead to the paradox that we can be healthy and not healthy simultaneously.

What is the way forward? It is tempting to ignore the problem – to carry on in the name of health regardless. And indeed this is what the great majority of 'health professionals' do at the moment. But although this is a natural response to conceptual difficulty, it is not an answer to it.

It is not merely a semantic problem, and nor is it practically trivial. It is a philosophical problem that requires philosophical investigation. And until it is satisfactorily answered by those who work in official health systems, massive problems of health policy, priorities and purpose, communication, professional–patient relationships and health care ethics will inevitably persist. It is only by coming to terms with the philosophical magnitude of the question 'what is health?' that practical progress toward clearer, more systematic and morally aware health work is possible.[5]

CHAPTER TWO

The Need for Philosophy

Many people see little point in a discipline whose first and sometimes only priority is to reflect on what things mean, yet there will always be a need for philosophy in our intellectual and social lives. If we never stand back to examine the relationship between our values and our actions how can we possibly assess the worth of what we do? For example, we have become so obsessed with 'making progress' – both as nations and as individuals – that we are in danger of losing the ability to ask what 'progress' really is. Fortunately, philosophy is an antidote to habit, convention and the blind pursuit of purely fashionable goals. Done with skill and integrity, philosophy can help us regain control over systems (like some clinical systems) that have come to operate in their own rather than in human interests.

We have been trying to answer the question 'what is health?', and have run into difficulties. It is as if we have stepped from what we thought was solid rock into a shifting quicksand. There are so many competing opinions about health that it looks impossible to decide which are sound and which are not. And it is in precisely this sort of situation that philosophical activity is required.

Philosophers are sometimes criticised for thinking in a vacuum. They are accused of abstracting ideas out of the practical world, and then playing trivial intellectual games with them. The charge is occasionally made against philosophy that there is no point in trying to work things out aculturally and ahistorically – that without the context of the real world any analysis must be meaningless.

Undoubtedly such criticisms are sometimes justified, but they are not always correct, and the converse can be criticised in turn. Never to take ideas out of the stream of practical life leads inexorably to a blinkered view of the world.

HOW CAN PHILOSOPHY HELP IN THE INQUIRY INTO THE NATURE OF HEALTH?

A full answer to the question 'what is health?' is possible only by standing back to take the widest possible view. This degree of detachment cannot be achieved by disciplines which traditionally favour one meaning or set of meanings of health. It is not that a social scientist will see only social factors affecting health, or that a biologist will see only biological factors. Rather, any specialist is bound by experience and training to regard certain factors as more pertinent than others, and will almost certainly be persuaded by her experience and expertise to describe and explain matters in a certain way.

SCEPTICISM ABOUT THE POWER OF PHILOSOPHY

The lack of direct involvement essential to philosophical investigation can be seen as a weakness. 'What does health have to do with philosophy?', it might be asked. It is usually taken for granted that health is the concern of practical people. It is generally assumed that health is something which is promoted, encouraged, prescribed for, or studied. It is achieved by behaviours and interventions such as exercise, moderation, good diet, drugs, and surgery. Health is the concern of the professionals who work at the sharp end of research and practice. Health is the goal of medics, biologists, psychologists, chemists, statisticians, nurses, and health educators. It may be a legitimate area of study for historians, sociologists, political scientists, economists, and geographers, but it is not the concern of philosophy.

Philosophers, it might be said, are expert at debating metaphysical issues (for instance, about different ways of classifying what can be known), proficient at resolving questions about what counts as genuine knowledge (for instance, deciding between what is known and what is merely believed), and they are authorities on assessing the validity of methods of inquiry (one aspect of logic). It is sometimes considered that the nearest philosophers can get to practical problems is in the field of moral philosophy, and that even then they are mainly interested in the production or discovery of basic moral rules (meta-ethics), so leaving the solution of particular ethical dilemmas to those who are most directly affected (it is still true, for example, that most 'ethics committees' do not include philosophers). The prevailing opinion is that philosophy should stick to its proper place and allow other specialisms to do the same.

Not everyone takes this view. However, those who do hold it do not understand what true philosophy is.

WHAT IS PHILOSOPHY?

As in all things, the following view of philosophy will not be shared by everyone.

PHILOSOPHY IS CLARIFICATION

The philosopher Ludwig Wittgenstein wrote:

> Philosophy aims at the logical clarification of thoughts.
> Philosophy is not a body of doctrine but an activity.
> A philosophical work consists essentially of elucidations.
> Philosophy does not result in 'philosophical propositions', but rather in the clarification of propositions.
> Without philosophy thoughts are, as it were, cloudy and indistinct: its task is to make them clear and to give them sharp boundaries. (p. 112)[6]

For Wittgenstein, philosophy ought to clear away confusion through the tightest possible analysis of words' meaning. But one should not expect philosophy to produce original ideas, and certainly should not expect philosophy to generate solutions to practical problems.

There is room for argument about Wittgenstein's conception of philosophy (which essentially holds that philosophers should merely point out philosophical errors). However, most philosophers would concur that philosophy must be opposed to dogmatism and single-minded ideology. Furthermore, those who undertake philosophy as a career would agree that true philosophy does not mean 'being philosophical' in the sense of resigning oneself to one's fate – rather it is the opposite. True philosophy does not mean 'having a general policy' – where there are acknowledged dos and don'ts – as is usually the case when people talk of the 'philosophy of management'. Nor is true philosophy the same as 'having a philosophy' in the sense of having a specific set of ideas. Philosophical activity is much more concerned with retaining the awareness that clarifications are incomplete than it is with obtaining 'the right answers'.

The tangible end-product of a philosophical labour can seem trite. It might result in a statement already known. It may have taken thousands of words to explain, but might apparently be said as well in a single sentence. It may even be that the end-product could have been arrived at by a less painful method. But if so then it would not be the same end-product, even though in isolation from the philosopher it would be identical in every respect.

Doing philosophy changes the philosopher. It demands an intense personal involvement with fundamental questions which cannot be let go and which must be pressed as far as possible. Philosophy involves asking questions (like 'what is health?') which perhaps seem too obvious to ask. Yet nevertheless a philosopher must ask them repeatedly and rigorously. Philosophy is a personal fight for clarity, a personal struggle – a wrestling match in which you are never certain that you have an opponent other than yourself. Philosophy is thus a process of self-education. It cannot be taught like language, science or geography, yet because it challenges and clarifies it can inspire philosophy in others. Philosophy is a process which develops a person. It is not something that can be passed on second-hand, although its results (books, papers, lectures) can.

CHILDREN ARE PHILOSOPHERS

We all have philosophical ability, but it seems that societies require obedience, persisting social structures and ordained law in order to function, and so philosophy is relentlessly kicked out of us. One of the many sad consequences of our inability to reconcile honest curiosity with good government is that we habitually dismiss the questions of children as 'childish questions', even though they are the questions of philosophers.

'What does God look like?', 'Why must I go to school?', 'Am I healthy?', 'What are raindrops?', 'Will I die?', 'Why is that lady so kind?', 'Why can't I wear trousers if I want to?', 'What does that word mean?', 'It isn't right that Susan can't afford to go on holiday, is it ?', 'Why do you say it's good to share, Daddy?', 'Why ... ?'

At first, we cannot help but try to dispel clouds with our inquisitiveness. Before we have grown to expect evasions and conventional answers ('that's just the way it is', 'we've all got to do it sooner or later', 'do as you're told') we are never satisfied. These sorts of question are honest. They stem from genuine puzzlement, and we should never stop asking them, however hard it gets and however much some of our fellow human beings would rather we didn't.

AN EXAMPLE FROM PLATO

Plato knew this, as the following illustration from *The Republic* shows.

The principal thread which runs through *The Republic* is the search for a definition of 'justice'. On the face of it 'justice's' meaning seems clear enough, but on analysis the issue turns out to be very complicated. Several definitions are suggested. Socrates squeezes out the sense and implications of each in order to test it for adequacy. At one point the question 'what is justice?' is cast in the form 'who is a just man?', and it is suggested that a just man is one who tells the truth and pays his debts. 'But is this so in all cases?', Socrates asks. For instance, should one return weapons to a madman?

Polemachus, his intellectual adversary at the time, responds:

> No, not in that case, not if the parties are friends and evil would result. He [Simonides – the original proposer of the idea] meant that you were to do what was proper, good to friends and harm to enemies.

But the view that justice does good to friends and harm to enemies will not do for Socrates, for several reasons. Among them is the fact that it is not necessarily the case that our friends are good and our enemies evil, and the observation that it is likely that if evil is rendered to evil people this will serve only to make them more evil still.

This debate about the nature of justice continues throughout *The Republic*. No final satisfactory definition is reached – and this in itself is an important lesson.

CONCLUSION

Philosophy is unique in its recognition that there are no questions which cannot or should not be asked, and that there can be no end to questioning. To do philosophy personal intellectual insecurity is a great strength if it is coupled with stubborn energy and patience. Where members of other disciplines reach answers with which they can be satisfied, at least temporarily, philosophers are personally compelled to force questions. However, this does not mean that a philosopher cannot produce a theory. Philosophy is not an affliction, nor is it a process which leaves no room for any other thought, but it does mean that a philosopher will never believe her theory to be a complete or final answer. She will criticise it and attempt to improve it as much as she can.

There are good reasons why we should all exercise our philosophical abilities, even if this involves shifting a lot of dust.

1.   We should all practise clarification if we want to grow. We should cultivate a systematic bloody-mindedness. We owe it to ourselves if we are thinking, autonomous people, not to accept any idea until we have thought it through personally.

2.   Where our work affects other people, as is the case with work for health, it is vital to recognise that not everyone has the same values and priorities. If we want to understand more about the world – and if we do not wish to colonise the minds of others – we must work to clarify other people's priorities, without imposing our own.

Questions like these should become habits:

What am I trying to do when I work to help people, and when I promote health? Does this person want what I regard as health? The chance of a few more weeks of life at the cost of hair loss and nausea may not be everyone's idea of a route to health, for example. Nor may stopping smoking at the cost of stress, family rows, and depression.

How am I influencing him? How can I tell what she wants? Is he capable of telling me? If not – if he is a young child or senile – how else can I find out? Such questions are both practical and philosophical, and can be answered only by combining both perspectives.

THE NEED FOR PHILOSOPHY – UPDATE

This chapter attempts to explain that the only way to get to the bottom of the question 'what is health?' is to practise philosophy. However, it contains a tension (at the time unnoticed) between **professional philosophy** and **philosophical thinking** (i.e. **philosophy as a form of thinking that everyone can and should do**).

This tension was a product of my situation as I wrote the first edition. I had just completed a largely happy six years as a student of philosophy in a British university philosophy department, during which time my mind had slowly been opened to a vast (and for me moving) history of philosophical inquiry. Naturally enough I associated philosophy with the thinking of the really notable philosophers whose work I had encountered: Aristotle, Descartes, Hume, Wittgenstein and others. I assumed (committing an error of induction my tutors would have jumped on had they realised) that all philosophy must be like this. However, as I struggled and failed to get a job as a philosopher, I began to realise that the world of university philosophy was just as closed and small-minded as most other professional institutions, and indeed that some philosophers (no doubt for reasons of self-preservation) were more concerned with belonging to the right philosophical school (being an Hegelian or a Wittgensteinian, being a Continentalist or an Analyst) than doing philosophy in the manner I had grown increasingly to cherish.

As a result the chapter defends two sorts of philosophy – **professional philosophy** and **philosophical thinking** – simultaneously and indistinguishably, when I was (and am) concerned only to advocate the latter.

Here is the unstated tension (remnants of which I have retained in this second edition): it is possible to be paid as a **professional philosopher** and yet never do any **philosophical thinking**, and *vice versa*. And – of course – it is also possible to be both a **professional philosopher** and a **philosophical thinker**.

Foundations was and is intended to advocate **philosophy as a form of thinking that everyone can and should do**. It is an appeal to the philosopher within each of us: if we want to answer philosophical questions (the sort that once came to us spontaneously as children) then we have to think philosophically – which means not taking anything for granted, eliminating inconsistencies, looking for or developing coherent patterns of meaning, and extending the logic of what we find into the practical world.

This view of philosophy is further than most contemporary professional philosophers would want to go. It is certainly much further than Wittgenstein thought appropriate. But then Wittgenstein lived in a world which valued ideas above all other things,[7] whereas I have made my way in an environment where practical results are usually all that matter. And Wittgenstein was wrong. Philosophy need not stop at clarification – in fact if a philosopher wishes to apply his understandings to the daily world, his best (and possibly only viable) option is to make the connections himself.

Let me restate my simple view of philosophy by briefly revisiting my own childhood. I can vividly remember a series of incidents in which I experienced the most intense feelings of frustration, surprise and disappointment, as my expectations and the reality of the adult world I would soon have to enter were unwantedly and unexpectedly rent apart. Most people will recall similar teenage episodes – in my case, being forced by my father to study chemistry instead of art, not being allowed to mimic the headmaster in a sixth form Xmas concert, having to study Latin in the absence of any reasonable explanation why – yet it is the earlier incidents that were the most telling for me (and I suspect for all of us). One in particular stands out, and epitomises the fight to retain philosophical ability.

I was about nine or ten and a junior school pupil, becoming known for precocious and provocative views (which I advanced in all innocence). One day the headmaster – Mr Blinkhorn – was conducting an English class and had marked me down for putting a comma before 'and'. I asked him in class why this was and he told me this was the rule – you couldn't put a comma before 'and' because this isn't allowed, it isn't the way to use 'and'. I naturally (literally it was in my nature) disagreed with him. I said the rule didn't make sense and that you could use a comma before 'and' because that way you could sometimes mean something different from not using a comma. But he wouldn't have it, and became increasingly annoyed with me. I knew, from past experience of either verbal humiliation or a backside slapping or both, how it would end if I persisted, so I took it as far as I dared and then shut up.

But I couldn't stop thinking about it and ended up working out all sorts of sentences with a comma before an 'and' (there are some in this book, and I still remember the 'Blinkhorn dictat' whenever I write one). I kept these to myself (there was no one to talk to about it anyway) and also had to deal with my puzzlement privately (unknowingly, I was undertaking an early 'wrestling match in which you are never certain that you have an opponent other than yourself'). I was truly torn – on the one hand here was this figure of authority telling me as a young boy that you definitely could not use a comma before an 'and', and on the other there was the clear evidence that you could and sometimes should. I knew I was supposed to accept what he said, and I even tried to – I don't think I used a comma before an 'and' for years afterwards. Yet I also knew he was wrong, not only about the comma but wrong – profoundly wrong – to dismiss my embryonic attempt to explore the art of writing.

Mr Blinkhorn was one of many people who have tried to destroy the philosophy within me. Somehow I held onto it, but most people aren't so fortunate. To do philosophy well – and to apply it to questions as complex as 'what is health?' – one needs more than childlike curiosity. One needs philosophical skills and techniques, experience, and knowledge of other philosophers' struggles with philosophical problems. Nonetheless it all depends on retaining the childhood philosophical instinct in the first place, on somehow protecting the ability to retreat from the pressures of the world to a quiet internal place to think freely.

Philosophy is basically a lifelong childhood rebellion and we should never forget it.

CHAPTER THREE

The Problem of Meaning

A prospective employer requests the opinion of a qualified physician on the present state of health of Mr Smith, a candidate for a job. Mr Smith is told that a physical examination is not required, but instead is asked some questions by the physician. The doctor asks about Mr Smith's 'general health'. Mr Smith replies 'it's fine'. The doctor asks about Mr Smith's diet, to which Mr Smith, thinking immediately of fried fish and chips and white bread and butter, assures the doctor that he has a 'healthy appetite'. The doctor inquires whether Mr Smith has 'a healthy social life too, with friends, exercise and conversation?' Mr Smith readily agrees, telling the doctor that he plays soccer every week. It does not cross his mind to mention that he suffers purgatory at each Sunday morning game as a result of Saturday night's eating and drinking excesses. Finally the doctor asks about Mr Smith's 'emotional state', to which Mr Smith replies that he is 'always happy' and has never been 'mentally ill'. The doctor is satisfied, and so are Mr Smith and his new employer.

This brief tale is sparse, hypothetical and ought to be implausible, but it is not impossible. Beneath its superficiality lie worrying misunderstandings – can a person who is 'always happy' really be 'mentally well'? – and a fundamental question: what, if anything, is communicated in encounters such as this, where words are used with little thought?

WHY SHOULD THERE BE SUCH DIFFICULTY IN PINNING DOWN THE MEANING OF HEALTH?

To understand why there should be such difficulty in pinning down the meaning of health it is important to recognise that the meanings of words can change over time, and that 'health' is not unique in this respect.

THE HISTORY OF THE WORD 'HEALTH'

Health has not always been considered the province of medicine. According to etymological dictionaries the word 'health':

OE hal, well, has derivative haelth (abstract suffix -th) -ME helthe-E health.[8]

is closely related to the word 'whole':

Main Entry: **1 whole**
Pronunciation: 'hOl
Function: adjective
Etymology: Middle English hool, healthy, unhurt, entire, from Old English hAl; akin to Old High German heil healthy, unhurt, Old Norse heill, Old Church Slavonic celu
Date: before 12th century
1 a (1): free of wound or injury: UNHURT (2): recovered from a wound or injury: RESTORED (3): being healed b: free of defect or impairment: INTACT c: physically sound and healthy: free of disease or deformity d: mentally or emotionally sound
2: having all its proper parts or components: COMPLETE, UNMODIFIED
3 a: constituting the total sum or undiminished entirety: ENTIRE b: each or all of the
4 a: constituting an undivided unit: UNBROKEN, UNCUT b: directed to one end: CONCENTRATED
5 a: seemingly complete or total b: very great in quantity, extent, or scope
6: constituting the entirety of a person's nature or development
7: having the same father and mother
synonym see PERFECT
– wholeness noun
synonyms WHOLE, ENTIRE, TOTAL, ALL mean including everything or everyone without exception. WHOLE implies that nothing has been omitted, ignored, abated, or taken away. ENTIRE may suggest a state of completeness or perfection to which nothing can be added. TOTAL implies that everything has been counted, weighed, measured, or considered. ALL may equal WHOLE, ENTIRE, or TOTAL.[9]

And this relationship is confirmed in the word 'hale':

Main Entry: **1 hale**
Pronunciation: 'hA(&)l
Function: adjective
Etymology: partly from Middle English (northern) hale, from Old English hAl; partly from Middle English hail, from Old Norse heill – more at WHOLE
Date: before 12th century: free from defect, disease, or infirmity: SOUND; also: retaining exceptional health and vigor synonym see HEALTHY.[10]

It is interesting to note the breadth of these ancient understandings. Health certainly used to have its modern meaning:

1 a (1): free of wound or injury: UNHURT (2): recovered from a wound or injury: RESTORED (3): being healed b: free of defect or impairment: INTACT c: physically sound and healthy: free of disease or deformity d: mentally or emotionally sound

But it could also quite properly mean:

2: having all its proper parts or components: COMPLETE, UNMODIFIED
3 a: constituting the total sum or undiminished entirety: ENTIRE...
4 a: constituting an undivided unit: UNBROKEN, UNCUT b: directed to one end: CONCENTRATED...
6: constituting the entirety of a person's nature or development

The latter understanding has been largely forgotten. As Michel Foucault notes, health's meaning shrank as professional medicine grew. 'Health' meant nothing more specialised than 'soundness of body, mind, and spirit' until about 200 years ago:

Generally speaking, it might be said that up to the end of the eighteenth century medicine related much more to health than to normality; it did not begin by analysing a 'regular' functioning of the organism and go on to seek where it had deviated, what it was disturbed by, and how it could be brought back into normal working order; it referred, rather, to qualities of vigour, suppleness and fluidity, which were lost in illness and which it was the task of medicine to restore. To this extent medical practice could accord an important place to regimen and diet, in short to a whole rule of life and nutrition that the subject imposed upon himself. This privileged relation between medicine and health involved the possibility of being one's own physician. Nineteenth-century medicine, on the other hand, was regulated more in accordance with normality than with health; it formed its concepts and prescribed its interventions in relation to the standard functioning and organic structure, and physiological knowledge – once marginal and purely theoretical knowledge for the doctor – was to become established...at the very centre of all medical reflexion. (p. 35)[11]

Foucault describes a gradual move from the notion that health is 'qualities of vigour, suppleness and fluidity' to the view that it is a state of biological normality which might be achieved by external intervention. Previously health was considered to be an autonomously created 'whole rule of life' rather than something which could be given by another person's intervention, independent of personal effort.

There has been a shift from an understanding of health as an ability to develop ourselves in accordance with our natures, to one that sees health solely as the absence of mental and physical defect.

FRANCIS BACON AND THE IDOLS

Francis Bacon understood the need for clarity and focus in human thought. He saw that human beings construct – involuntarily, through carelessness, and sometimes even deliberately – certain barriers against understanding. He described these unfortunate habits as akin to the worship of 'Idols' or false gods. He identified four types: 'Idols of the Tribe', 'Idols of the Cave', 'Idols of the Theatre', and 'Idols of the Market-place'.

Bacon used the expression 'The Idols of the Tribe' to refer to the human tendency to suppose that our senses give full and accurate knowledge of reality, and that the order we perceive in nature actually exists. Bacon considered this tendency a fault, arguing that human perceptions are 'false mirrors' on reality, distorting the information we receive from the external world.[12]

'The Idols of the Cave' are the particular prejudices of each human being, our personal biases which have resulted from our unique experiences, friends, teachers, political views, religious beliefs, and so on. The evidence we receive of external events is always interpreted or adulterated in the light of these Idols. According to Bacon:

...every one (besides the errors common to human nature in general) has a cave or den of his own, which refracts and discolours the light of nature; owing either to his own proper and peculiar nature; or to his education and conversation with others; or to the reading of books, and the authority of those whom he esteems and admires....[13]

Evidence can never be purely received – for it to mean anything to an individual it has to be interpreted, and this act of interpretation creates what are often wrongly described as 'objective facts' (see 'the formula' in *Health Promotion*[14]).

The 'Idols of the Theatre' cause the errors which:

> ...have immigrated into men's minds from the various dogmas of philosophies.[15]

Here Bacon was describing the folly and intellectual stagnation which he believed had been produced by an unthinking adherence to the doctrines of Aristotle, but he was also making the general point that blind acceptance of 'received wisdom' is an empty and destructive obedience.

The most powerful 'Idols' of all are those which still plague us to the highest degree. They are the 'Idols of the Market-place' (which appear in abundance whenever health issues are discussed). These 'false notions' arise from the 'exchange and commerce' of words. Many politicians, journalists and academics, amongst others, worship the 'Idols of the Market-place' with regrettable fervour.

Bacon identified two main problems arising out of the 'worship' of these Idols. Firstly many words are ambiguous. Often two people talk at 'cross-purposes' – they use the same word with a different meaning and fail to realise their mistake. Secondly, words are apt to be taken to represent things, even though these 'things' do not actually exist. Certain words (which in fact stand for nothing concrete) are thought to refer to real entities, just because they are written or spoken so frequently. Bacon's examples were 'fortune' and 'prime mover'. 'Mind' might be a further example and so might 'health'.

Solzhenitsyn has explained Bacon's thesis in a powerful way:

> All right, then, let's call it a more refined form of the herd instinct, the fear of remaining alone, outside the community. There's nothing new about it. Francis Bacon set out his doctrine of idols back in the sixteenth century. He said that people are not inclined to live by pure experience, that it is easier for them to pollute experience with prejudices. These prejudices are the idols...
>
> What are the idols of the theatre?
>
> The idols of the theatre are the authoritative opinions of others which a man likes to accept as a guide when interpreting something he hasn't experienced himself... sometimes he actually experienced it, only it's more convenient not to believe what he's seen.
>
> I've seen cases like that as well...
>
> Another idol of the theatre is our over-willingness to agree with the arguments of science. One can sum this up as the voluntary acceptance of other people's errors!... Finally there are the idols of the market-place.
>
> This was easiest of all to imagine: an alabaster idol towering over a swarming crowd in a market-place.
>
> The idols of the market-place are the errors which result from the communication and association of men with each other. They are the errors a man commits because it has become customary to use certain phrases and formulas which do violence to reason. For example, 'Enemy of the people!' 'Not one of us!' 'Traitor!' Call a man one of these and everyone will renounce him...
>
> And over all idols there is the sky of fear, the sky of fear over-hung with grey clouds.

> You know how some evenings thick low clouds gather, black and angry clouds, even though no storm is approaching. Darkness and gloom descend before their proper time. The whole world makes you feel ill at ease, and all you want to do is to go and hide under the roof in a house made of bricks, skulk close to the fire with your family.[16]

When Solzhenitsyn writes of the 'herd instinct, the fear of remaining alone, outside the community' he could be describing the fear of philosophy, the fear of resisting the easier answer, the fear of thinking for oneself. This fear is calmed by skulking close to accepted views, by adopting the opinions of others without making searching personal assessment, and by hiding behind verbal smokescreens.

Bacon's comments about the 'Idols of the Market-place' become obvious as soon as one makes a serious attempt to understand the meaning of words which do not have straightforward ostensive definitions. These words have more than one meaning – they have *meanings*.

WORDS CAN BE SMOKESCREENS

If we have only a vague idea of what we mean by a word, if we have only a hazy recognition of a word's possible range of meanings but have never made the personal effort to clarify them, certain words can act as 'verbal smokescreens'. In Bacon's words they become 'barriers against understanding', making clear communication and full understanding impossible. Smokescreens can occur accidentally or be created deliberately by those who wish to conceal deeper issues (continual praise of the 'health service' by some politicians is a typical example) but the effect is the same: visibility is decreased, or even reduced to nil.

RAYMOND WILLIAMS AND KEYWORDS

Raymond Williams listed a group of familiar words which have more than one meaning. Not all words are of this type. We can agree what is meant by words such as 'typewriter', 'library', or 'stethoscope', but some words – such as 'rationality', 'democracy', 'justice', and 'health' for instance – seem to be the source of continuing misunderstandings and disputes. Williams called these words 'keywords'.

Williams argued that disputes over the correct meaning of keywords can reveal the depth of underlying issues, though substantive disagreements cannot be resolved only through the investigation of words' meanings:

> On the contrary, most of the real issues [remain] however complete the analysis, but most of them ... [cannot] really be thought through, and some of them ... cannot even be focussed unless we are conscious of the words as elements of the problems. (p. 14)[3]

In Williams's opinion the correct use of these words is not simply a matter of training. To believe only one use of a word is correct is a brittle confidence. Williams admits that if language is to be used at all it must depend on the confidence that words do have right meanings – or else everything would be permanently equivocal, and this would be clearly impractical – yet for Williams the question of meaning must be faced, at least periodically. If not the result will be a false clarity of definition – where once one definition has been selected from a range of possibilities that definition is insisted upon, thus screening the actual range of meanings (and the substantive issues) with an illusory clarity.

EXAMPLES OF KEYWORDS

Democracy

One of the most confusing and abused words Williams discusses is 'democracy'. It is so often used as a rhetorical bludgeon. Williams puts the problem succinctly:

> No questions are more difficult than those of *democracy*, in any of its central senses. Analysis of variation will not resolve them, though it may sometimes clarify them. To the positive opposed senses of the socialist and liberal traditions we have to add, in a century which unlike any other finds nearly all political movements claiming to stand for *democracy* or *real democracy*, innumerable conscious distortions: reduction of the concepts of *election*, *representation* and *mandate* to deliberate formalities or merely manipulated forms; reduction to the concept of *popular power*, or government in the *popular interest*, to nominal slogans covering the rule of a bureaucracy or an oligarchy. It would sometimes be easier to believe in democracy, or to stand for it, if the nineteenth-century change had not happened and it were still an unfavourable and functional term. But that history has occurred, and the range of contemporary sense is its confused and still active record. (pp. 86–87)

Rationality

The words 'rational' and 'rationality' also have more than one meaning. In some cases these meanings are incompatible. The true nature of rationality is disputed, although most people agree that it is a characteristic that human beings should be proud of.

People are described as rational if they are efficient in the pursuit of their chosen goals, or if they are logical, or if they are sensible, or if they are reasonable and realistic. These meanings are each different, though the main conflict is between the first and last two combinations – between the idea of a 'rational person' who is logical and efficient above all else, and the idea of a 'rational person' who is reasonable and sensible above all else.

It is not difficult to imagine cases where these different ideas of rationality clash to such an extent that it becomes difficult – if not impossible – to say that both people are being rational. For example, '**rational person A**' might be pursuing the goal of bringing about policy changes designed to deprive 80% of the members of a society of all wealth, power, and voting rights. He might be pursuing this goal with great logic and efficiency – he might be a brilliant politician, logician, and legal expert. '**Rational person A**' might be opposed by '**rational person B**' who is trying to be fair and reasonable, and who is against the sort of ruthless extremism displayed by '**rational person A**'. She might be concentrating on promoting ideas of natural justice and balance, and may consider her preference to be the truly rational option.

Are both people rational?

GALLIE'S SUGGESTION THAT ALL LEGITIMATE MEANINGS OF WORDS MUST SHARE IN AN HISTORICAL TRADITION

The philosopher of history, W. B. Gallie, argues that certain concepts are 'essentially contested'. Certain words, he claims, have meanings which people with different sets of values will never be able to agree on.

Gallie goes further than Williams. He claims that each concept must possess some historically based core of meaning recognised as part of the concept by all who use it. In Gallie's words:

> ...the adequate understanding of such concepts involves some appreciation of their history. At the very least we must accept that every proper contestant use of such a concept can be traced back to a commonly acknowledged exemplar, and can be justified on the ground that, and to the extent that, people can be found who regard it and can rationally defend it as the best possible development of the original exemplar's aims.[17]

There is much in what Gallie says. In order to have any worthwhile conversation about the meaning of a word it must be possible for the discussants to have some common ground. For example, in the case of democracy all democrats – whatever their particular interpretation of democracy – must be egalitarian in some sense. In the case of art, debaters will need to find a piece of work they both agree is an example of art or else they will not have a shared point of reference. However, there are two problems with Gallie's argument:

1. Words do not necessarily have undisputed historical meanings. As Williams has pointed out – and as we have seen in the case of 'health' and 'whole' – meaning depends at least as much on the current ways a word is used than on an appeal to an ancient definition.

2. Gallie's suggestion merely pushes the controversy back a degree. Instead of dispute about the legitimacy of particular meanings the argument centres on the question: which is the true exemplar? Williams comes nearer the truth when he shows that words are often used with a variety of meanings, some of which may be contradictory, without there necessarily being any point of agreement recognised by the protagonists – though this does not rule out the possibility that there may be a hidden common factor.

AN EXAMPLE OF HOW PHILOSOPHY CAN CLARIFY MEANING

In the following section the contestable words 'definition', 'theory', 'concept', and 'conceiving' are discussed, not least since they are frequently used in writing about the nature of health, usually in a confused and confusing fashion.

DEFINITION, THEORY, CONCEPT, CONCEIVING

Definition

A definition is a specific, fixed label designed to indicate one meaning of a word or a phrase. A definition can be either a single word or a set of words. A definition is impersonal and must be communicable. Definitions are important in that they provide initial footholds towards understanding, but they should never be thought of as 'the last word' since all definitions include theories of one kind or another, and theories change over time. The dividing line between definitions and theories is fuzzy.

Theory

A theory is designed to explain more than a definition. A theory can be articulated publicly or held privately. Theories aim for consistency externally and internally. That is, theories are intended to be consistent with features outside their own structure, they are designed to explain, and cannot be self-contradictory if they are to be plausible.

Karl Popper and Michael Polanyi agree that theories, formulated in language and made public, are no longer part of the inventors of those theories. Polanyi, for example, argues that a theory on which a person relies is unaffected by any fluctuations which occur within that person. He says:

> A theory is something other than myself. It may be set out on paper as a system of rules...it is not I but the theory which is proved right or wrong when I use such knowledge...A theory cannot be led astray by my personal illusions. To find my way by a map I must perform the conscious act of map-reading and I may be deluded in the process, but the map cannot be deluded and remains right or wrong in itself, impersonally.[18]

Theories are necessary for reasoned understanding and they allow practical changes to be made to the physical world. This is not the place to discuss the range and types of theory. The point to note is that it is possible to express theories independent of the theorist.

Concept

Concepts are often thought to be vague and nebulous. The 'concept of health', for example, is commonly supposed to contain elements which have something or other in common, the precise nature of which is forever unclear. People discuss 'cluster concepts' as if concepts were huge, shapeless umbrellas sheltering related ideas. Rock groups used to write 'concept albums' when they had a vague idea that they wished to explain something quite complicated through their music, or when all their songs seemed to have links. Used in these ways the word 'concept' is used to justify imprecision. The nature of health is not clear so health is referred to as a 'concept', but this is cowardice. It is ducking the issue. To say that health is a many-faceted 'cluster concept' does not help us understand either what we are thinking or trying to do. To use the word 'concept' in this way actually imposes a (sometimes convenient) barrier to further thought and clarification. It can be an excuse for sloppy thinking.

Happily, there is a better way to understand the meaning of the word.

Concepts must be held personally because they involve an essential personal element based on feeling, experience and memory. Concepts can be described externally, although not without residue.

Personal concepts are unique, will be ambiguous and will contain various meanings. Concepts are not personal theories since they do not aim to be consistent, and involve more than theory. Theories might be part of personal concepts, and parts of concepts might be developed into impersonal theories.

Concepts are not innate in a person but develop as a result of interplay between conceiving, theory and practice. Neither are concepts inherent in nature. There is no such thing as *the* concept of health. Concepts are not 'out there', independent of human beings, waiting to be discovered.

In the literature, 'the concept of health' is always either a particular theory of health or a collection of theories of health. What is meant, for example, by 'the/a concept of health as the absence of disease' is a crude theory that health involves the absence of disease. But this is to misuse the idea of a 'concept'. It is not putting forward a concept to say that 'disease is a biological imbalance in a normally hierarchically harmonious arrangement of cells, tissues, and organs', it is the beginnings of a theory.

In fact a concept can never be fully articulated. Concepts are held personally. A person's concept of health could involve the thought that disease must not be present, but must involve more than this to be a concept. It will involve memory, recollections of diseases experienced, of times when no disease was present (if this ever was the case), of happiness, of comfort, of waking up feeling that one could take on the world (perhaps). It will also involve the constant interplay between personal conceiving and changing circumstance. This personal element cannot be translated without residue. What a person feels and thinks about his concept can be described – at which point part of the concept becomes an articulated theory – although a lot must remain which cannot be put into words.

The theory of a concept is never the same as the concept. It will probably have become considerably more consistent as a result of the translation.

A Problem

Could a person possess a concept of health which made reference to anything he chose, however ridiculous? For instance, could a person possess a concept of health which involved the theories that health is undesirable, equivalent to suffering, that health is indicated by the colour blue, that health involves the creation of impediment, and so on? The person would be conceiving, and might be onto something which would ultimately culminate in an impersonal theory. However, as it stands his concept is *impotent*, and this is an important distinction. To be powerful a concept must have *external relevance*. Other people must be able to understand what the concept means in theory or practice, or both. Other people must be able to see the point of it.

Not any collection of ideas can count as a concept of health because the *potency* of a concept depends upon an interplay between conceiving, consensus, articulation, illustration, and physical states of affairs. A potent concept's sense must be transmittable through theory and practice to other people. Furthermore, to be meaningful, to be more than a collection of unconnected individual ideas, a concept must have an identifiable focus or subject area.

Examples of Concepts

People's concepts of 'evolution' and 'mind', for instance, involve theories, examples, personal experience, analogy, imagination and personal puzzling, whether we realise it or not. Within each concept the theories, examples and imaginings may not be fully compatible with each other. For example, some people's concepts of evolution take account of Darwin's theory, neo-Darwinian variation of this theory, Creationist counter-claims, gaps in the fossil record, theories of chance and determinism, school biology lessons, personal opinions about plausibility, and so on – usually in an incomplete and disorganised fashion. Similarly, people's concepts of mind may take account of theories about the nature of the brain and the correspondence between patterns of electrical activity and patterns of thought, behaviourism, personal experience of dreams, déjà vu, dualism, Descartes' thought, the 'soul', religion, spirituality and perhaps countless other aspects of life.

Even 'simple' concepts, such as concepts of colours, smells, sounds and so on, cannot be divorced from personal experience. I have an image of a red amaryllis but I cannot imagine red in the abstract. It is always a ribbon, or paint on canvas, or chalk on a wall, and so on (this is a disputed position in professional philosophy – see Hilary Staniland[19]).

Conceiving

This is the capacity that enables us to form concepts and theories. It permits choice, decision, and assessment. It is the basic ability by which we understand anything. Conceiving occurs frequently; conceiving is the act of assessing, weighing up, entertaining ideas, playing with inconsistencies, appealing to personal experience, fitting theories with perceived states of affairs, and inventing analogies. Theorising is a deliberately specific and logical part of the act of conceiving.

Arthur Koestler's book, *The Act of Creation*, gives a fascinating account of how we come up with solutions to problems for which no specific rules have been given. He argues that such situations are remarkably common. The key is not held only by people of genius who can somehow come up with an entirely new idea. This is a mythical notion. The key to a new perspective is synthesis, and synthesis can take place only when thinkers are able to escape rigid rules to conceive more freely:

> When life presents us with a problem it will be attacked in accordance with the code of rules which enabled us to deal with similar problems in the past. These rules of the game range from manipulating sticks to operating with ideas, verbal concepts, visual forms, mathematical entities. When the same task is encountered under relatively unchanging conditions in a monotonous environment, the responses will become stereotyped, flexible skills will degenerate into rigid patterns, and the person will more and more resemble an automaton, governed by fixed habits, whose actions and ideas move in narrow grooves.

He may be compared to an engine driver who must drive his train along fixed rails according to a fixed timetable.

Vice versa, a changing, variable environment will tend to create flexible behaviour patterns with a high degree of adaptability to circumstances – the driver of a motor car has more degrees of freedom than the engine-driver. But novelty can be carried to a point – by life or in the laboratory – where the situation still resembles in some respects other situations encountered in the past, yet contains new features and complexities which make it impossible to solve the problem by the same rules of the game which were applied in those past situations. When this happens we say that the situation is blocked . . . A blocked situation increases the stress of the frustrated drive. What happens next is much the same in the chimpanzee's as in Archimedes' case.

When all hopeful attempts at solving the problem by traditional methods have been exhausted, thought runs round in circles in the blocked matrix like rats in a cage. Next, the matrix of organized, purposeful behaviour itself seems to go to pieces, and random trials make their appearance, accompanied by tantrums and attacks of despair – or by the distracted absent-mindedness of . . . single-mindedness; for at this stage – the 'period of incubation' – the whole personality, down to the unverbalized and unconscious layers, has become saturated with the problem, so that on some level of the mind it remains active, even while attention is occupied in a quite different field . . . until chance or intuition provides a link to quite a different matrix, which bears down vertically, so to speak, on the problem blocked in its old horizontal context, and the two previously separate matrices fuse . . . The creative act is not an act of creation in the sense of the Old Testament. It does not create something out of nothing; it uncovers, selects, re-shuffles, combines, synthesizes already existing facts, ideas, faculties, skills. The more familiar the parts, the more striking the new whole. Man's knowledge of the changes of the tides and the phases of the moon is as old as his observation that apples fall to earth in the ripeness of time. Yet the combination of these and the other equally familiar data in Newton's theory of gravity changed mankind's outlook on the world.[20]

Theorising is the process of choosing the most appropriate elements from one's concept of one or more subjects, refining, rejecting, and assessing for consistency, explanatory power, and simplicity. The forming of a theory is a personal activity which draws on the fullest range of human abilities. It is logically distinct from calculating, which is a process which can be specified precisely, and which machines can be programmed to do more efficiently than can people.

Personal conceiving is a prerequisite for defining and theory invention, and is ultimately necessary in order that decisions can be made about the worth of competing theories. Conceiving transcends theory, paradox, and inconsistency. It permits judgement between theories without reliance on further theory. Conceiving allows a person to cope with the simultaneous existence of alternative and conflicting possibilities, whereas definitions and theories have a more limited focus. Conceiving is never static but is a liberating quality since it allows people to cope with change and unique situations.

Conceiving is not entirely language dependent. It is also dependent on unspecifiable human factors which stem from experience of life. It is not the case that two human beings – who will inevitably have had different experiences – possessing knowledge of exactly the same theories will necessarily make the identical decisions in identical circumstances. Judgement is part of conceiving, and this aspect cannot be fully captured in words and symbols. The development of concepts and theories demands judgement at all stages, and this judging does not rest only on theory possession. It is not enough to know how to recite a theory, a person must know why he is reciting it, and what this means and implies.

◆

The above discussion has (I hope) shown how making the effort to clarify can be illuminating. Writing on health often uses these words, almost always ambiguously, and sometimes with meanings different from those offered above. Whatever the case, knowledge of this clarification will enable a reader to understand more easily the intentions and thoughts of the various authors.

The results of this brief clarification are used in **Chapter Eight**.

SUMMARY AND CONSOLIDATION

1.   This chapter has explained the extent of the problem of meaning. The problem is not only confined to discussions about health, but affects a wide range of keywords. Philosophical activity can help dispel much of the confusion.

2.   'Health' is a word used with a variety of meanings. Which particular meaning is used seems to depend on the context, the user, or both these factors.

Everyone involved with health in any way should attempt a personal clarification of the meaning of the word. Everyone should practise philosophy, in other words. It is not enough to read this book. The arguments and problems must be thought through and addressed personally.

3.   Given that 'health' is a word which is used with a variety of meanings it should be possible to identify various schools of thought about its meaning. If the arguments of Williams and Gallie are correct then each school will understand health to have a particular meaning or range of meanings dependent on the values held by the members of that school.

4.   In Gallie's opinion it should be possible to identify an historical tradition which links all the preferred meanings to an initial exemplar. This is perhaps asking too much. However, it should be possible to discover a contemporary uncontested general sense of health – an idea which is an essential part of all the meanings of health and about which no one would disagree. If the idea of health is not to be meaningless – if the word 'health' is not to mean anything one wants it to mean – then it must be possible to display some limit to the sense of the word.

THE PROBLEM OF MEANING – UPDATE

The second part of this chapter is probably the most esoteric in the book, and I can understand why some readers might prefer to skip it and get on with exploring the different theories of health explained in **Chapter Four**. However, the discussion about definitions, theories, concepts and conceiving was included in the first edition for reasons which still hold:

1.   These words – particularly 'concept' used in the phrase 'concept of health' – abound in the health literature and can and do act as 'verbal smokescreens'. However, once one understands that concepts are:

> ...ambiguous and will contain various meanings. Concepts are not personal theories since they do not aim to be consistent, and involve more than theory. Theories might be part of personal concepts, and parts of concepts might be developed into impersonal theories...

then one can judge more clearly whether or not this is what other authors mean by 'concept'. And if they mean something different it is possible to contrast readily any alternative meanings with the meaning expressed above.

2.   What could be more appropriate, in a chapter devoted to the problem of meaning, than to assess the most basic units of meaning themselves – the forms of thought we use to understand, categorise and discuss the world around us?

3.   It is argued that a concept is too vague to be a theory, but can be the precursor of a theory, given sufficiently deep and energetic theorising.

4.   Definitions and theories are explicit and public, and it is definitions and theories (not concepts) of health that we need if we are to make theoretical and practical progress.

5.   The discussion of theories and concepts is an integral and important part of the book's structure – and should help readers understand more of **Chapter Five** in particular, in which a concept of health (my own) is tentatively developed into a definition and a theory, exemplifying the processes described above.

6.   The discussion is part of an argument for conceiving, and therefore for **philosophy as a form of thinking that everyone can and should do**. The whole book makes the case for independent thinking about the nature of health and the practical task of health work. If health workers are to be able to break free of the chains of convention to develop a workable, broader understanding then they must understand both what it is to conceive, and how important it is to allow oneself to conceive.

For further clarification:

Definition
A specific, fixed label designed to indicate one meaning of a word or a phrase.
Definitions provide initial footholds towards broader understanding.

Theory
A theory is designed to explain more than a definition.
Theories aim for consistency with what they are trying to explain, and consistency within their account of themselves.
Theories are necessary for reasoned understanding and help us make systematic practical changes to the physical world.

Concept
Concepts must be held personally because they involve an essential personal element based on feeling, experience and memory.

Personal concepts are unique, will be ambiguous and will contain various meanings. Concepts are not personal theories since they do not aim to be consistent, and involve more than theory.

Theories might constitute part of personal concepts, and parts of concepts might be developed into impersonal theories.

Conceiving

The elusive capacity that enables us to form concepts and theories.

The act of assessing, weighing up, entertaining ideas, playing with inconsistencies, appealing to personal experience, fitting theories with perceived states of affairs, and inventing analogies and metaphors.

Theorising may be part of conceiving, but it is not all of it – it is the deliberately specific and logical part of the act of conceiving.

A summary of the elements of definition, theory, concept and conceiving

Note that 'conception' is used in the **Introduction** to indicate a way of graphically displaying possible ways of conceiving of health.

Finally, the discussion of the relationship between 'health' and 'wholeness' (expanded in this second edition) should not be overlooked. The history of the word health is included in **Chapter Three** to show that words' meaning can shift over time – and to show that exactly this has happened to 'health', with the consequence that the word is particularly prone to interpretation. Furthermore, the demonstration that health is traditionally associated with 'being a whole person' is important to the book in general because:

1.   It sets the scene for the development of the **foundations theory of health**, which is true to the venerable, rounded understanding offered in Old and Middle English dictionaries.

2.   It shows that our modern, automatic view that medicine is the root of health care is neither objectively true nor necessary. We used to have different understandings of health and we can have them again if we want to.

CHAPTER FOUR

Theories of Health

INTRODUCTION

This chapter discusses four theories of health, and various ways of working for health based on them. Each theory has been distilled from a wider collection of theories that seem to group together, and is intended to represent their core. The result is partly artificial – other analysts could choose (and have chosen – see Kovacs[21]) different groupings and themes. Nevertheless, the present clarification offers sufficient theoretical progress to enable the construction of the more comprehensive understanding of health advanced in **Chapter Five**.

CLARIFICATION

DISEASE AND ILLNESS

Something must first be said about the words 'disease' and 'illness'. It will come as no surprise that it is impossible to define these 'keywords' to everyone's satisfaction. It is, however, possible to propose a reasonably clear distinction between them.

Concerned that these and associated words are used too loosely, the philosopher–physician team of Bernard Gert and Charles Culver analysed their meaning:

> In the English language a cluster of words are used to refer to the conditions that concern us here. Three of the most important are 'disease', 'illness', and 'injury', but there are many more: 'wound', 'disorder', 'defect', 'affliction', 'lesion' and 'disfigurement', to list a few. While these terms have distinct though partly overlapping connotations, which can be fairly precisely identified, there is nevertheless an arbitrary element in the labelling of the various conditions... An interesting example of the arbitrary nature of this labelling is the condition experienced by deep sea divers who return from the depths too quickly. It is referred to as either 'caisson disease' or 'decompression illness', while essentially all of the associated ill effects are due to the cellular injury caused by nitrogen bubbles forming in the various bodily tissues. (p. 65)[22]

For medical science the identification of disease depends on measurement and comparison against normal states. Typically the process evolves from the description of a few unusual cases, to the description of a general 'disease pattern' (called a syndrome) for which the cause is not clear, to the delineation of a specific condition with a known cause. Early in the history of medicine the identification of disease, and the ways of distinguishing one disease from another, depended solely on the sorts of signs and symptoms reported and presented externally. As techniques developed, the diagnosis and understanding of disease began to rest on the underlying tissue changes, and now hinges mainly on biochemical analysis. In each case what was and is described as a disease is a pattern of factors which have occurred in sufficient people for a specific type of deviation from a particular norm to be identified.[23]

Given the above, it is commonly supposed by those who diagnose disease that a satisfactory definition of the word exists. Yet according to Culver and Gert this assumption is incorrect. They discuss a number of attempts, and dismiss most as woefully inadequate. For example they quickly find fault with a definition offered in William White's book, *The Meaning of Disease*.[24] In White's opinion:

> Disease can only be that state of the organism that for the time being, at least, is fighting a losing game whether the battle be with temperature, water, micro-organisms, disappointment or what not. In any instance, it may be visualised as the reaction of the organism to some sort of energy impact, addition or deprivation.[24]

Culver and Gert conclude – bluntly and correctly – that on this definition one wrestler held down by another is suffering a disease. They also condemn a definition found in a standard pathology textbook as being similarly vague and all inclusive. According to Peery and Miller:

> Disease is any disturbance of the structure or function of the body or any of its parts; an imbalance between the individual and his environment; a lack of perfect health.[25]

Culver and Gert comment ruefully that this offers three separate, equally poor definitions. Clipping nails, puberty, and being tied to a chair are all diseases according to the first definition. The second is too vague to be useful, and the third is circular: it merely says that having a disease is to lack perfect health, and that people lack perfect health when they have a disease. The question of what a disease actually is remains untouched.

Culver and Gert go on to discuss more acceptable definitions, preferring those which refer to *deviation from a norm for a species, biological disadvantage*, and *medical disorder intrinsically associated with distress, disability, or certain types of disadvantage*. They offer their own definition of a 'malady' which incorporates the above 'cluster of words'. However, as far as a definition of disease is concerned, they accept a proposal (put forward by Lester King) which incorporates both the notion of a range of evils, and also the idea that deviation from a norm is a necessary condition for disease:

> Disease is the aggregate of those conditions which, judged by the prevailing culture, are deemed painful, or disabling, and which at the same time, deviate from either the statistical norm or from some idealised status. (p. 197)[4]

There are those who would find fault with this definition, since it combines the notions of 'disease' and 'illness' which they would rather think of as separate. For example, David Field, a sociologist, argues that 'disease' refers (or should refer) to a medical conception of pathological abnormality indicated by a set of signs and symptoms, while 'illness' refers (or should refer) primarily to a person's 'ill-health' and is indicated by *feelings* of pain and discomfort.

Field takes the view that illness can be the result of pathological abnormality, but pathological abnormality does not necessarily cause illness. A person can feel ill without medical science being able to detect disease. For instance, a person can feel 'under the weather', be depressed, feel alienated, be in pain, and be in despair, without the presence of recognised disease. Conversely, a person can have no symptoms of illness and yet be diseased. For example, cervical cancer can be detected by a smear test without the patient being aware of any discomfort, and teeth can decay without causing pain. Disease, on this understanding, is a measurable abnormality while illness is experienced as a quality, and we cannot measure our feelings in the way we measure physical states.[26]

Field's distinction is part of a protest – advanced by thousands of academics over the last thirty or so years – against medicine's myopia. The claim is that since disease relates to the organic level (according to the currently accepted view) and illness to the psychological and social level, by focusing almost total attention on disease, scientific medicine does not pay the heed it should to all aspects of sickness. A person's psychological reaction to his disease is often neglected, even though it might be the most important part of the experience for the individual, and even though attention to it might assist a cure.[27] Moreover, it can be detrimental to believe that diseases and illnesses can always be distinguished, because disease and illness are events which happen to complete human beings. What's more, some diseases/illnesses do not fall neatly into one category or the other. For example, it is not clear whether alcoholism should be considered a disease or an illness. Nor is it obvious how to classify a person who has a significant allergy but no current symptoms.

SUMMARY

Diseases can be thought of as certain sorts of abnormality that occur in physical bodies. These abnormalities can be identified by medical science. Illnesses are feelings people experience. It is important to make this distinction because 'disease' and 'illness' are often used interchangeably when they should not be. People 'feel ill', they do not necessarily 'feel diseased'. A person cannot be ill without feeling it but a person can be diseased without feeling it. Furthermore, while some diseases can be infectious, illnesses cannot.

Medicine works to control and eradicate disease, and in so doing sets out to beat illness. However, some aspects of ill-health are not the province of medicine. These illnesses may have a range of causes against which medicine has no defence.[28] Yet by habitually conflating the words 'disease' and 'illness', the medical profession gives the impression of greater power and scope than it actually has.

The chart displays four distinct types of theory: the theory that **health is an ideal state**; the theory that **health is a level of fitness necessary to perform normal tasks**; the theory that **health is a commodity** which may be bought or given, gained or lost; and the theory which holds that **health is a personal strength or ability**. The four types

A Simplified Summary of Theories of and Approaches Designed to Increase Health

Theories of Health

The theory that health is an ideal state

– A goal of perfect well-being in every respect.
– An end in itself.
– Disease, illness, handicap, and social problems must be absent.

The theory that health is the physical and mental fitness to do socialised daily tasks (i.e. to function normally in a person's own society)

– A means towards the end of normal social functioning.
– All disease, illness and handicap which disable normal functioning must be absent.
– Chronic illnesses, diseases and handicaps can be present.

The theory that health is a commodity that can be bought or given

– The rationale which underlies medical practice.
– Usually perceived as an end for the provider, a means for the receiver.
– The more disease, illness, pain and injury, the poorer the health of the patient.
– Health may be restored piecemeal, through therapies offered by distinct specialisms.

A group of theories which hold that health is a personal strength or ability – either physical, meta-physical or intellectual

– These strengths and abilities are not commodities, and cannot normally be given or purchased. They may exist innately, or they may be developed by individuals on their own, by individuals working together, or by individuals receiving support from others. These strengths and abilities can also be lost.

Approaches Designed to Increase Health

The sociological approach

– Concerned with a range of factors that influence health, for good or bad. Commonly works to describe unequal distribution of disease and illness, and the unequal use of health services by different sections of society. Tries to explain the causes of these inequalities. Typically uses its descriptions and explanations to provoke social reform and greater equality.

The approach of medical science

– Emphasis on clinics, hospitals, biology, statistics, and measurement of pathological conditions against normal standards.
– The causes of disease and the effects of drugs and surgical techniques are researched to increase understanding and to allow preventive, curative and educational measures.

The humanist approach

– Regards health as a goal to be achieved personally. Disease, illness and other problems may co-exist with health.
– Recognises that people are complex wholes living within, and permanently influenced by, a constantly changing world. Recognises (and accepts as real) interconnections between the physical, the spiritual and the intellectual.
– Recognises a latent capacity for self-development in all human beings who have the actual or potential ability to understand the implications of their actions.

Common Factor

The provision of the conditions necessary for the achievement of some biological and chosen potentials, and of conditions which enable people to work towards the achievement of other biological and chosen potentials, is the overall goal of all approaches. The provision of suitable conditions can be thought of as the removal of obstacles to human potential.

have elements in common. For instance, to varying degrees, disease, illness, handicap, and pain must be absent in three of the four theories. Furthermore, all theories, except the theory that **health is an ideal state** can, again to varying degrees, be described as being both a means and an end.

It is possible to devise compatible combinations of the theories. For example, gaining health thought of as a commodity could enable a person to function normally in society, this normal functioning could be seen as evidence of a personal strength and might also boost a person's ability to cope. What's more, the combination of these states could be what the individual in question would describe as ideal. However, in-depth examination of the theories makes it clear that they can also be incompatible. For instance, the theory that health is an ideal state is not normally consistent with that of health as normal functioning since few people would seriously claim every aspect of their present function as ideal, indeed many of us would argue quite the opposite. Health as normal functioning is not necessarily consistent with the theory that health is strength since such strengths are often created at times when normal functioning is disrupted, and it is possible for strength to exist regardless of considerations of normal functioning. In addition, the theory that health is a commodity is, in many circumstances, opposed to health as strength since commodities are given or purchased and health as a strength or ability to respond positively can be seen as a task which requires personal or collective effort.

To some extent the theories are compatible, and to some extent they are not. Sometimes the theories and approaches aim at the same target, at other times they set their sights differently.

Note too that the boxes shown on the chart are neither fixed nor watertight. People's thoughts about health are usually complex and vary from context to context. People rarely have one set opinion about health, rather they draw on elements of different theories (derived from all manner of formal and informal sources: academia, TV, gossip, folklore and so on) to create their personal concepts. Similarly, the various approaches designed to increase health do not make use of just one theory. At least some of those who adopt a particular approach can recognise the merits of other theories, just as they can recognise the value of other approaches. The point of presenting a simplified model of such a complicated area is the same as that of this book as a whole: to make things clearer so that we know where we stand, and to enable us better to identify the implications of thinking seriously about health.

THEORIES OF HEALTH

THE THEORY THAT HEALTH IS AN IDEAL STATE

Theories which hold that health is an ideal state – a state of supreme well-being – seem always to have been a part of human dreams. Our own age is no exception. The World Health Organisation (**WHO**) offered this famous definition of health in its *Constitution* of 1946:

> Health is a state of complete physical, mental and social well-being and not merely the absence of disease and infirmity.

In one important respect this definition is commendable, since its intention is to show that health involves more than not being infirm and not having a disease. However, the stated aims of **WHO** are admirable and yet hopelessly idealistic (see **Theories of Health – Update** below for a comment on **WHO**'s actual aims). The thinking (presumably) is that the target might as well be set as high as possible – although it won't be achieved, the higher it's set the higher the actual achievement will be. Cast like this the ambitions seem noble, yet they are fatally undermined by the fact that the proper basis for them – rigorous theoretical clarification of their meaning – has not been established. As they stand the **WHO** definition and theory are little more than well-meaning rhetoric: totally comprehensive and so totally meaningless (they may also act to disguise other intentions).

What Is Wrong with this Definition and the Theory which Inspires It?

1.   Although the definition states (correctly) that health is more than 'the absence of disease and infirmity', it presupposes that a person cannot be healthy if she has any kind of physical or mental disease, illness or infirmity. It even assumes that a person cannot be healthy if he happens to be suffering from a social problem of any sort. Furthermore, in describing health as an absolute, **WHO** sets up a single, ideal standard. But to set such a standard condemns most – in fact almost certainly all – human beings to the rather disheartening belief that each of us is inevitably and permanently unhealthy.

2.   The definition (and **WHO** as a whole – see **Theories of Health – Update**) does not face up to the many controversies about what the phrase 'complete physical, mental and social well-being' might mean. The meanings of the terms 'physical well-being', 'social well-being' and 'mental well-being' are all disputable. Choices about what 'states of health' conform to these notions are bound to depend on the values of the people who make them. For example, social well-being in a kibbutz is a different state from social well-being in a new development of 'executive homes' in a leafy English suburb. In the suburb a person's state of social well-being could hinge on whether he possesses two cars or a mere one, whereas social well-being is achieved by sharing resources within the community in a kibbutz.[29] Which condition is true social well-being? Which is the ideal? Is it possible to say?

There are similar difficulties with the other phrases. For instance, in the USA an ambitious, successful, egoist business woman would probably be described as having mental well-being so long as she was not psychiatrically unwell, but in a communist country such a state of mind could be (and has been) taken as a mark of a sickness.[30]

Furthermore, it would be perfectly possible for a person to put forward an argument that her mental well-being depends on her being able to write and distribute racist literature. If she found such activity necessary, fulfilling and it made her happy it would be difficult to argue that her practice did not contribute to her mental health. The trouble is (a) that not everyone will agree that the racist author and publisher actually does have mental well-being, and (b) her racist activities could harm the mental well-being of other people. Consequently, if 'health for all' means that every member of the human race must have mental well-being then (as a matter of logic) 'health for all' will never be achieved whilst the mental well-being of different individuals is in conflict (and this seems an inevitable part of the human condition).[31]

3.   The third problem is that although it may be an inspiration for some to have such a supreme personal and global goal to aim at, it can mislead others into striving for something that cannot possibly be attained. And this can sometimes deflect people from more realistic goals and lines of development.

In an influential work on the nature of health, René Dubos[32] has explained that the belief in ideal health is a useless mirage which continues to draw people fruitlessly on. Dubos argues that contemporary dreamers either refer back to an imagined era in which 'ideal health' was universally achieved, or anticipate a utopian future. He explains that what he calls 'tribal memories' can become transmuted into mythical recollections of idyllic happiness experienced in a 'golden age', and that the future hope for people in the present is offered by what he calls 'the magic bullets of medicine' (if only the right treatment for our ills could be found, if only real 'miracle drugs' would become available, 'ideal health' could be reclaimed or achieved at last). And this – Dubos contends – is a myth that seriously distorts our understanding of health.

4.   To talk of 'ideal health' as if it is an absolute, specifiable, definable state is a mistake. It is as meaningless and useless as asking for a description of a 'perfect human being'. What would such a person be like? Would such a person be male or female; 5, 20 or 65; black, white or yellow; an athlete, an intellectual, a comedian; a miner, a poet or a bank manager? People have different bodies, ages, backgrounds, and talents – obviously the optimum state of existence for each of us will vary according to how and what we are.

5.   There are senses in which an individual might have an ideal state of health, though such a state would probably be experienced only occasionally and fleetingly. However, there is another sense in which it is not possible for any person to have 'ideal health'. This is if health is thought of as the maximum fulfilment of *all* the potentials of a particular individual. Such a state cannot be achieved because we all possess more latent potentials than we can ever fulfil. Choices are made throughout a person's life about which direction to take, about which potential to develop and about which potentials will have to lie dormant. At school choices are made about whether to specialise in mathematics, technology, science, the arts, or art and design. Such specialisation continues to be forced on us because we simply have far too many options to fit into our short lives.

Furthermore, some latent potentials cannot be realised simultaneously because they would be in conflict. For example, an obsessive pursuit of business goals would leave no room for voluntary work overseas, although both potentials might have been latent in an individual.

The Implications of Applying this Theory

There is little more that can be said about the implications of this theory – it is theoretically incoherent and therefore impractical.

THE THEORY THAT HEALTH IS THE PHYSICAL AND MENTAL FITNESS TO PERFORM SOCIALISED DAILY TASKS

The American sociologist Talcott Parsons advocates this theory. In Parsons' opinion health is:

> ... the state of optimum capacity of an individual for the effective role and tasks for which he has been socialized.[33]

This definition is part of a wider theory (about the way human societies function) too complicated to be discussed properly here. But this is not a great disadvantage since Parsons' theory of health makes sense removed from its wider context.

Parsons' idea is that health is the standard of physical and mental function necessary for a person to perform the activities expected of him, according to the norms of the society in which he lives. At first sight this seems a plausible way of thinking about health, so long as one is content to regard health and disease as opposites: people who are diseased or ill are often unable to continue normally.

On Parsons' theory a person cannot be described as healthy if she has a disabling disease or illness. Parsons does not consider the possibility of degrees of health. Instead he considers health an 'optimum capacity' – anything less cannot be health for Parsons.

If a person is no longer able to function normally he will adopt the 'sick role'. According to Parsons, if individuals adopt this role they can claim the right to be excused from their normal social duties, but are also obliged to seek the medical advice of friends, relatives, and healers since they have a duty to get better.

What is Wrong with this Theory?

1.   It describes health too narrowly. Health is conceived as the polar opposite of disease and illness, and so disease and illness become the only health problems which interfere with a person's capacity to perform the tasks for which he has been socialised. Yet health is – as we shall see in the next chapter – logically more than the antithesis of disease and illness, and theories which fail to recognise this are inevitably incomplete.

2.   The theory is unappealing to those, such as the World Health Organisation, who regard health positively. Parsons' theory sees health as a state which must be achieved in order to continue as before. It makes sense when applied to individuals who are happy with their lives, who enjoy their work, and who are achieving and developing along ways of their choosing, but it falls down in cases where the 'role and tasks for which he has been socialized' are unstimulating. A person's role and tasks might even

be part of a counter-productive process. It can be that working in a physically or mentally stressful, or monotonous, job – or never having worked at all – is precisely what causes individuals to adopt the 'sick-role' in the first place. For illustration, consider the work of coal miners, workers on building sites, and business people working long hours under high levels of stress. Miners often develop diseases of the lung as a result of years of exposure to coal dust; tradesmen and labourers in physically demanding jobs are often injured and tend to 'fade out' as their physical strength dissipates with age, and business people can suffer such problems as excessive drinking and heart disease at an early age as a result of their jobs. In cases such as these advocates of the 'health as normal functioning' theory must face a tricky question: how does it make sense for a person to work for, or be assisted towards, a return to a state of health (that is, the state of 'optimum capacity of an individual for the effective role and tasks for which he has been socialized') when that state must eventually contribute to a state which the theory must describe as ill-health?

3.   If an alternative account of health is preferred the deliberate refusal or inability to continue normally need not be a sign of mental or physical illness, but a healthy desire for change.

The Implication of Applying this Theory

To work for health in this sense is to work to maintain societies in their present states.

THE THEORY THAT HEALTH IS A COMMODITY

The predominant image of health care in today's increasingly Westernised world is that health is a commodity – something which can be bought, given, sold or lost. Many of those who see health like this believe people are naturally healthy, and would remain so were it not for untoward outside influences. On this view, given normal luck and normal circumstances people remain healthy, but just as someone can lose a wallet so we lose health when abnormal circumstances pertain.

The belief that health is a commodity has arisen inexorably from the approach of medical science, and is equally compatible with capitalism. According to it, health can be supplied piece by piece, if necessary without any effort from the recipient. The idea is that health can be purchased just like everything else tangible can be purchased, for example by buying surgery or drugs to cure a person's heart disease. The possession of the drug is thought to bring health with it. Conceived in this light health seems independent – somehow outside people – something to be captured (usually at the commercial rate) given the right procedure.

To sum up, there are three main elements to this theory. Firstly, on this understanding health tends to be thought of as an ideal goal which might be recaptured given the right sort of medical intervention. Secondly, health is thought to be a commodity apart from individuals (something which can be *added on* to a person by the use of drugs, physical therapy, exercise, 'health food' and so on). And thirdly, health can be bought and sold just like any commodity, and is subject to precisely the same market laws as any other merchandise.[34]

These three themes combine in subtle ways.

What Is Wrong with this Theory?

In a sense the theory is very plausible. Certain conditions have to be fulfilled, certain things have to be provided, in order to create some aspects of health. And it is unquestionably true that many of the commodities offered by medicine can improve health.

However, what most concerns opponents of this theory is the idea that health can be thought of as a commercial object. For example, Oliver Sacks, a well-known neurologist and writer, acknowledges that the approach of medical science has advantages, but argues that it is insufficient to solve problems regularly encountered in work to increase health. Sacks claims that a true physician must be both an artist and a scientist. He describes medicine as a 'romantic science' – a vocation which needs laws, algorithms, procedures and mechanisms, but which also requires empathy, personal communication, non-verbal understanding, and intuitive emotional interaction. Sacks rejects the idea of health as a commodity because it ignores these artistic aspects – after all, he argues, a machine can dispense drugs and information – and also ignores the fact that human beings are unique, indescribably complex wholes. Sacks says:

> ...we pretend that modern medicine is a rational science, all facts, no nonsense, and just what it seems. But we have only to tap its glossy veneer for it to split wide open, and reveal to us its roots and foundations, its old dark heart of mysticism, magic and myth...
>
> There is, of course, an ordinary medicine, an everyday medicine, humdrum, prosaic, a medicine for stubbed toes, quinsies, bunions and boils; but all of us entertain the idea of another sort of medicine, of a wholly different kind: something deeper, older, extraordinary, almost sacred, which will restore to us our lost health and wholeness, and give us a sense of perfect well-being.
>
> For all of us have a basic intuitive feeling that once we were whole and well; at ease, at peace, at home in the world; totally united with the grounds of being; and that we lost this primal, happy, innocent state, and fell into our present sickness and suffering. We had something of infinite beauty and preciousness – and we lost it; we spend our lives searching for what we have lost; and one day, perhaps, we will suddenly find it, and this will be the miracle, the millennium. (pp. 26–27)[35]

Sacks believes that the search for our 'lost health' through the acquisition of commodities is a misguided quest which unfortunately is sometimes encouraged by the apothecary or physician. Instead Sacks thinks of health as personal fulfilment, whether a person's chosen goal is happiness, a sense of reality, a feeling of being fully alive, or whatever is personally fulfilling. 'This basic metaphysical truth', as Sacks describes it, can be:

> suddenly twisted (and replaced by a fantastic, mechanical corruption or falsehood). The chimerical concept which now takes its place is one of the delusions of vitalism or materialism, the notion that 'health', 'well-being', 'happiness', etc. can be reduced to

certain 'factors' or 'elements' – principles, fluids, humours, commodities – things which can be measured and weighed, bought and sold. Health, thus conceived, is reduced to a level, something to be titrated or topped up in a mechanical way. Metaphysics in itself makes no such reductions: its terms are those of organisation or design. The fraudulent reduction comes from alchemists, witchdoctors, and their modern equivalents, and from patients who long at all costs to be well. It is from this debased metaphysics that there arises the notion of a mystical substance, a miraculous drug, something which will assuage all our hungers and ills. (p. 28)[35]

By seeking to offer health only as a commodity, and by holding out the false hope of an effortless return to 'ideal health', medical science conceals our wider potentials from us, because it undermines our unique 'metaphysical' (spiritual and intellectual) strengths.

THE GROUP OF THEORIES WHICH HOLD THAT HEALTH IS A PERSONAL STRENGTH OR ABILITY

This group of theories can be united under a humanist banner. Here is what the British Humanist Association has to say about humanism:

What is Humanism?

It is difficult to provide a single definition of Humanism, since Humanism is not a set doctrine or dogma and Humanists are, by definition, freethinking individuals.

Humanists do not believe in god or heaven, but in the power of science, reason and human experience to make sense of our lives. Humanism represents the positive affirmation of our humanity based on a rational belief and behaviour which includes the views that this life and this world are all we can truly know, that there are no supernatural beings or forces and no sacred beings or texts and that our values and morality must come from within ourselves and our experience, rather than from above.

Humanists hold that the most important factor in all our thoughts and actions is our shared membership of the human race, and that it is up to us to make the best of our time together here...

Humanism is an approach to life based on reason and our common humanity, recognising that moral values are properly founded on human nature and experience alone.[36]

Whether or not a person is diseased, ill, or suffering is ultimately immaterial to the humanist view of health. Sometimes these states are necessary in order to allow an individual to grow, although in general the humanist thinks of them as obstacles to be eliminated if possible. Humanism believes people should be helped to develop themselves by the removal of impediment by any means, including the means offered by medical science.

As we saw from Sacks' criticism, to regard health only as a commodity is to miss matters of fundamental importance to human existence. As an alternative, this group of theories argues that health is either an unquantifiable resilience or an ability to adapt positively to the inevitable problems and sufferings life throws up – it is not something that disappears in the presence of disease and illness. Rather health is a way of responding appropriately, in all the ways open to human beings, not only the biological ones.

Health is thus a means towards further and greater ends – if a person can resist or adapt positively to problems of different kinds then she has a position from which she can develop her potential to the fullest. Of course, this strength and ability to adapt positively can often be a significant and difficult end to be achieved in itself.

This group of theories purposely returns us to the position we began to lose in the eighteenth century – where health was thought of holistically. According to these theories health is once again not something which can be precisely defined. It is a way of living – a 'whole rule of life'.[11]

THE THEORY THAT HEALTH IS A METAPHYSICAL STRENGTH – THE POINT OF VIEW OF OLIVER SACKS

It is important to understand the unusual experiences that shaped Sacks' deeply held beliefs, otherwise it will be unclear why he is so passionately convinced of the existence of a deep and unquantifiable human strength. Sacks claims to have witnessed an awesome 'spiritual health' in his work with patients suffering from an array of debilitating mental and physical handicaps. He has described many bizarre, frightening, and yet inspiring case histories of a fascinating group of patients in *Awakenings*.[35]

This book is important for several reasons, the most compelling of which is that despite enduring the most extreme disabilities Sacks' patients fought back however they could: their human spirit could not be drowned in spite of everything. The concomitant tragedy (though Sacks does not make this explicit) is that this spirit can be totally concealed in countless people living normal lives.

Sacks' book describes the lives and reactions of the few survivors of 'the great sleeping-sickness epidemic' (encephalitis lethargica) of 60 years ago, and at the same time shows the implications of their struggles. Of particular interest is how the patients responded to the so-called 'miracle-drug' L-DOPA (*laevo-dihydroxyphenylalanine*). The euphoric reaction to the arrival and promise of this drug incited Sacks to a vehement attack on 'medical magic'. Although the immediate effects of L-DOPA were often dramatic, 'awakening' many people from years of immobility, the drug failed to restore sufferers permanently, and often caused worse illness than the original disease – although on balance Sacks feels that L-DOPA should be described as beneficial.

Sacks explains that the 1916–17 winter in Vienna saw the start of a 'new' disease which spread worldwide over the next three years (a viral cause was eventually identified). At a very rough estimate 5 million people died or were ravaged by the sickness. No two patients ever manifested the same picture. The most frequently occurring set of symptoms was somnolent illness followed by Parkinsonian effects. (Parkinson's disease is a syndrome of symptoms with 'festination' prominent. Sufferers will experience hurriedness of steps, movements, words, and thoughts, with the feeling that this hurry is not caused by their own volition.)

The pandemic raged for 10 years, to disappear in 1927. A fairly common pattern was that a sufferer would experience severe, comatose sleep or equally severe insomnia, but after a period of time, whilst the virus was still at large, a sufferer could recover to some extent only to experience Parkinsonian effects. Sacks states that over a third of the sufferers died during the initial stage of the sleeping sickness, either in states of coma so deep as to preclude arousal, or in states of sleeplessness so intense as to preclude sedation:

> Patients who suffered but survived an extremely severe somnolent/insomniac attack of this kind often failed to recover their original aliveness. They would be conscious and aware – yet not be fully awake; they would sit motionless and speechless all day in their chairs, totally lacking energy, impetus, initiative, motive, appetite, affect or desire; they registered what went on about them with profound indifference. They neither conveyed nor felt the feeling of life; they were insubstantial as ghosts, and as passive as zombies. They were ... awaiting an awakening which came (for the tiny fraction who survived) fifty years later. (pp. 14–15)[35]

Sacks points out that approximately 500 'positive' disorders have been noted. Among the most common he lists akinesia (total lack of movement – the inability to make voluntary movements), aphonia (the inability to make sounds), aphrenia (the stoppage of thought), and akathisia (the inability to keep still, an intense urge to move, restlessness or fidgets to a most extreme degree). Some patients could be 'living statues' for days and even for years on end. Some could speak, some:

> ... showed automatic compliance or 'obedience', maintaining (indefinitely and apparently without effort) any posture in which they were put or found themselves, or 'echoing' words, phrases, thoughts, perceptions or actions in an unvarying circular way ... Other patients showed disorders of a precisely antithetical kind ... immediately preventing or countermanding any suggested or intended action, speech or thought: in the severest cases, 'block' of this type could cause a virtual obliteration of all behaviour and also all mental processes – such constrained catatonic patients ... could suddenly burst out of their immobilized states into violent movements or frenzies. (p. 17)[35]

Patients also displayed a wide spectrum of 'tics' (spasmodic twitches of the facial muscles) and compulsive movements at every functional level – yawning, coughing, sniffing, gasping, panting, breath-holding, staring, glancing, bellowing, yelling, and cursing. Nearly half the survivors became liable to extraordinary 'crises', in which they might experience such effects as an almost instantaneous attack of Parkinsonian symptoms, catatonia, tics, obsessions, hallucinations, 'block', increased suggestibility or negativism, or even a simultaneous combination of these disorders. These crises would last for a few minutes to hours before disappearing as suddenly as they had appeared.

The point of explaining a little of the detail of these unfortunate people's great suffering is to give an idea of the extent of their disability, which nonetheless could not completely hide their spirit, desires, and potentials from a person of Sacks' obvious sensitivity. He was frequently overwhelmed by the impression of a tremendous inner strength in his patients which even the most severe difficulties could not extinguish. Sacks believes this spirit is neither a product of his imagination nor a manifestation of the illness, but a quality which actually exists, driving people to continue to develop in the face of apparently insurmountable odds.

'Miriam H.' was a patient of Sacks who during her long illness suffered violent furies, apathetic depression, and crises in which she was morose and was compelled to look up at the ceiling. Miriam was partially paralysed and chair-ridden. She was given three courses of L-DOPA and always responded well at first, but twice had to have the treatment discontinued because of the occurrence of severe crises. Her third treatment was a relative success in so far as she learnt to control her crises and showed 'a clear-cut if unspectacular therapeutic response'. Sacks writes of her:

> ... all in all, Miss H. has done well – amazingly so, considering the existence she has led. Against all odds, Miss H. has always managed to be a real *person* and to face reality without denial or madness. She draws on a strength unfathomable to me, a health which is deeper than the depth of her illness. (p. 128)

THE THEORY THAT HEALTH IS A RESERVE OF PHYSICAL AND MENTAL STRENGTH

The collection of theories which hold that health is a personal strength or ability has received support from sociological inquiries into the 'health beliefs' of 'ordinary people'. Independent research projects into 'lay concepts of health' show that non-health professionals typically think of health as a reserve or stock of strength. Indeed, this view is held by people of at least three distinct cultures (by Mexican peasants, by middle-class Parisians, and by elderly Aberdonians).

Mexican peasants speak of people with a 'stock of health' as possessing 'sangre fuerte' (strong blood).[37] The Parisian study, conducted by Claudine Herzlich,[38] relied on interviews with 80 middle-aged and middle-class respondents. She encountered at least three concepts of health. The first was 'health in a vacuum', which was seen as a state without illness and regarded as an impersonal, all-or-nothing fact. The second was the idea of a 'reserve of health'. This was said to be robustness – a capacity to resist the assaults of illness or injury (a personal characteristic which may vary over the years). The third was health as 'equilibrium', which was to do with physical well-being, good humour, good relations with others, activity, and the assimilation of disorders.

The Aberdeen study discovered that people able to withstand bouts of illness were popularly thought to have 'reserves of health', while people who had 'lost their health' were considered 'done' or 'washed out'. The researcher, Rory Williams, found that the elderly people he interviewed felt that 'health' could be lost completely or partially but might be recovered, and that 'weakness' – the opposite of 'health' – could also fluctuate. This weakness is not necessarily disease, more a proneness to be ill.

Williams' interviewees could be accused of some illogic (for example they seemed to regard health as 'absence of disease' and also believed that disease can exist without compromising good health). Nevertheless, the idea that 'health is strength' clearly has a real and everyday meaning for people – not merely a meaning constructed by academics. Williams writes:

> That health is something more than the absence of disease has been suggested by the notion of good health as the power of overcoming disease which is actually present. To

this may...be added the complementary notion of bad health as the loss of such power even when disease is absent.[39]

Williams' report shows, unsurprisingly, that 'lay-people' think of ourselves as wholes:

> ...though health is thus sometimes the absence of serious disease, it is also possible to refer to someone as healthy even though serious disease is said in the same breath to be present.

> The meaning of this conjunction of health or strength with disease was most clearly illuminated by my informants in accounting for a severe crisis which had been surmounted and which had ultimately proved transitory. A brother was described as 'the strong one of the family': his leg was amputated because of gangrene, he was put into 'this sort of glasshouse they put you in', he actually died and was resuscitated, and though he was never expected to come up out of this illness – he did. People who were well, strong, fit or healthy had the power to 'come through' or 'come up'; and hence they could also declare that they had always been healthy despite a list of sicknesses and diseases which was often alarming.

> Hence although health can be used simply to mean the absence of disease, it is also used in a far more complex and positive sense; and this positive sense often dominated discussion by my samples of the relation of health to activity and moral effort.[39]

(For more on lay understandings of health see also **References 39–43**.)

THE THEORY THAT HEALTH IS AN ABILITY TO ADAPT

This theory has strong links with the other two in this group, and draws on points already discussed, yet it also has its own identity. Versions of it have been put forward by writers such as Katherine Mansfield, René Dubos and Ivan Illich.[32,44,45]

Both Dubos and Illich urge a reduction in medical science's influence, because its emphasis on clinical technology impedes our ability to adapt autonomously. Part of their case is that improved health (meaning here a decrease in the prevalence of disease) has come about mainly as the result of social measures designed to correct the ills of industrialisation, to provide better nutrition, better housing and better work conditions – it has not arisen exclusively or even primarily through laboratory science. The practical achievements of the nineteenth-century reformers did not come from a biochemical understanding of medical problems. Laboratory science advanced human understanding by discovering the complex world of germs and nutrient balances, but practical improvements came as a direct result of improved hygiene and sanitation. Dubos writes:

> The time has passed when explorers on land or at sea have to depend on heavy loads of lemons and animal food in order to protect themselves against scurvy and other deficiency diseases. A few small packets of synthetic vitamins can now make an adequate diet out of proteins, carbohydrates, fats, and water. A dash of chlorine and an effective filtration bed will make any water supply more typhoid-proof than the most sparkling streams brought from high mountains...

> But while modern science can boast of so many startling achievements in the health fields, its role has not been so unique and its effectiveness so complete as is commonly claimed. In reality...the monstrous spectre of infection had become but an enfeebled shadow of its

former self by the time serums, vaccines, and drugs became available to combat microbes. Indeed, many of the most terrifying microbial diseases – leprosy, plague, typhus, and the sweating sickness, for example, had all but disappeared from Europe long before the advent of germ theory. (p. 19)[32]

Dubos goes on to make the point that other maladies, such as cancer, vascular disorder, and mental disease, which were not affected by the sanitary movement, remain problems. He suggests that the causes of these ills may be directly related to modern life (he implicates pollution and excessive competition), which does not allow man sufficient time in which to adapt.

Dubos's argument is cast against the theory that health is an ideal state. He points out that this utopia cannot be achieved because of the constantly changing nature of existence, and neither should it be desired since we are adaptable creatures who can live and flourish in almost any Earth environment. Dubos claims that the capacity to explore, create and face the dangers and challenges of new environments is an essential human characteristic, and that to define one way of life alone as 'healthy' (which is a possible consequence of an arrogant interpretation of abstract general definitions of health[46]) is unacceptably autocratic.

Dubos does have faith in the potential of the scientific method to discover the causes of disease, and to suggest remedial procedures, but this is not the whole story of health. He says:

> Whether concerned with particular dangers to be overcome or with specific requirements to be satisfied, all the separate problems of human health [Dubos seems to mean disease here] can and eventually will find their solution. But solving problems of disease is not the same thing as creating health and happiness...Health and happiness are expressions of the manner in which the individual responds and adapts to the challenges that he meets in everyday life. And these challenges are not only those arising from the external world, physical and social, since the most compelling factors of the environment, those most commonly involved in the causation of disease, are the goals that the individual sets for himself, often without regard for biological necessity. Nor can the problem be usefully stated [sic] by advocating a return to nature...Harmonious equilibrium is an abstract concept with a Platonic beauty but lacking in the flesh and blood of life. It fails, in particular, to convey the creative emergent quality of human existence...The Garden of Eden, the Promised Land that each generation imagines anew in its dreams, and all the Arcadias past and future could be sites of lasting health and happiness only if mankind were to remain static in a stable environment. But in the world of reality places change and man also changes. Furthermore, his self-imposed striving for ever-new distant goals makes his fate even more unpredictable than that of other living things. For this reason health and happiness cannot be absolute and permanent values, however careful the social and medical planning. Biological success in all its manifestations is a measure of fitness, and fitness requires never-ending efforts of adaptation to the total environment which is ever-changing. (pp. 22–25)[32]

WHAT IS WRONG WITH THIS GROUP OF THEORIES?

1.   They are all too vague. The natures of the strengths and abilities referred to are not specified (though to be fair to the theorists in question, they point out that it is a mistake to attempt such precision). However, for practical purposes it is not at all clear what the 'metaphysical strength' discussed by Sacks is, nor is it obvious what a

person's 'reserve of strength' is. The meaning of the phrase 'health is the ability to adapt' seems straightforward at first sight, but without details about what the possession of such an ability involves it is impossible to orient health work toward its achievement.

Unless the advocates of this view give more substance to their theories it will remain legitimate to argue that such responses as insanity, larceny, suicide, murder, megalomania, and apathetic depression are positive adaptations to external circumstances. They are certainly adaptations and – if they can be justified by some as being 'positive' – in the absence of a comprehensive list of approved inclusions and exclusions, count as positive examples they must.

2.   Because of this vagueness, because of this sugar-coating of ambiguity, people who wish to work for health as adaptation are given few guidelines about how to select and achieve targets for intervention. In order to increase health, whether it is thought of as strength or as the ability to adapt, health workers must have a good understanding of the types of element which constitute 'strength and ability', in order to encourage these in those who lack them.

THE IMPLICATIONS OF APPLYING THIS GROUP OF THEORIES

If the elements of people's lives relevant to their reserves of strength and their abilities to adapt could be specified more clearly, then the implications for practical health work would be great. The current vogue of regarding medical care and health care as synonymous would pass out of fashion to be replaced by the idea that it is people's abilities to cope and to take full charge of their own lives that are the most important features of work for health. Instead of maintaining health centres staffed almost entirely by medics and para-medics, such places would offer a more comprehensive service.

APPROACHES DESIGNED TO INCREASE HEALTH

THE SOCIOLOGICAL APPROACH

Social scientists of various sorts have produced a great deal of valuable research which shows that a person's social class, work, and standard and style of living can affect his lifespan and the sorts and severity of disease and illness he is likely to suffer. *Inequalities in Health: The Black Report*,[47] written by a group chaired by Sir Douglas Black, President of the Royal College of Physicians, provides extensive information about the ways in which class differences are associated with differences in 'health'. This, and a host of similar research reported regularly in health and social care journals,[48] indicates that people's chances of avoiding such diverse problems as back pain, injury, depression, diabetes, epilepsy, bronchitis, kidney disease, heart disease, and cancer demonstrably improve according to their wealth and social position.

Problems

Social research is vital. It produces – amongst a lot else – a stream of information that argues for itself that the world's social systems do not treat a great number of people fairly and equally, that social injustice can produce physical and mental problems. However, the approaches joined under the heading 'the sociological approach' suffer from two problems:

1. There has been insufficient analysis of the meanings and sense of the word 'health', and not enough notice taken of the scope of the various theories of health. Ample evidence of this can be found in most sociological journals concerned with medicine, illness, and health.

2. This means that although sociologists constantly point out that health is much more than a target for medicine, and is inevitably a political issue, they do not make the further step of acknowledging that health is more than the opposite of disease and illness. To put the issue crudely, many sociologists think of health like this:

Health *————————* Disease and Illness

where health is achieved when disease and illness are absent. Like misnamed health services around the world, sociology is still primarily concerned with the causes of illness and disease – believing that if all of these could be eliminated then full health would follow – than it is with the question of what health really is and how this can be achieved. A book by Jeanette Mitchell, *What Is to be Done about Illness and Health?*[49] is typical in this respect. The author asks such questions as: What is the nature of the connection between the work we do, the money we earn, where we live, how often we get sick, and the kinds of illnesses we suffer? Where do the chronic illnesses, heart attacks, cancers, and handicaps come from? Why do some people get them and others not? How can we account for the present pattern of illness and death, with its stark class contrasts? Is all this illness inevitable? What is the medical system doing to remedy the problems we face? Could medicine and health be different?

She then offers interesting and informative answers to these questions. She makes the point that:

> There could be less chronic and recurrent illness. Our problems are less a matter of biology than politics. Better health is possible. (p. 41)

However, while she recognises that health is a wide-ranging issue influenced by many factors and of interest to many diverse professions, she cannot let go of the simplistic equation that not being ill must be the same as being healthy. She points out that the now classic definition of health offered by the World Health Organisation (see p. 42) is rather mystical, but she does not think the issue has to be complicated. She says:

> ...what we want is not really hard to grasp. We want fewer chronic and recurrent illnesses, less cancer and heart disease, less depression and anxiety. Of course we cannot

hope to abolish illness, but the important point about the class pattern of health and illness... is that it is evidence of how much unnecessary ill health most people face. The level of health presently enjoyed by the people at the top of British society should not be seen as an absolute standard, but it is at least an indicator of how much better our health could be if our lives were different... the top civil servants [have] a quarter the rate of heart attacks of men at the bottom of the Whitehall hierarchy; [there is] twice the level of chronic illness among people in social class five compared with social class one; levels of chronic depression among working-class women [are] five-times greater than among middle-class women. That's a lot of unnecessary illness we could do without. (pp. 213–214)

This writer, and social science in general, is concerned with a central aspect of the problem of how to achieve health. Social science has shown that membership of social classes 4 and 5 (as they are described in the UK at least) is an obstacle in itself, and can create further unnecessary obstacles such as disease and illness. By displaying the problem social science works to remedy it, but this is not the full story. Social science in general fails to acknowledge that a person can be ill, diseased or handicapped and yet still enjoy a reasonable degree of health.

THE APPROACH OF MEDICAL SCIENCE

Western medicine espouses a scientific approach designed to increase health conceived as the opposite of disease. The clinical approach has well-known characteristics, most of which have been the subject of widespread criticism in recent years. These criticisms have not been properly digested by the medical establishment.

Assumptions of Medical Science

Though the following are generalisations – and not all doctors subscribe to every one of them – they nevertheless reflect the tone of contemporary medical culture. Medicine's central assumptions are:

1. *That health occurs when disease is absent.*

2. *That health is a commodity.*
The medical approach favours the theory that health is a commodity. This idea is energetically encouraged by the medical industry which supplies the drugs and the technology (for evidence, see the advertisements in any of the trade magazines). It has (controversially) been argued that the purpose of medicine within a market economy is primarily to match this supply with a demand that medicine is partially responsible for creating.

The left-wing academic Andre Gorz has, for example, made the point that:

> Fundamentally... the practice of medicine is a business. The relations between medical professionals and the public are market relations. The professional sells what the patients ask for or are willing to buy individually.[50]

Inequalities in individual health are explained by pointing out that different social groups have unequal access to medical products (which is one of the gripes of the sociological approach described above). This sort of thinking furthers the myth that society has a supply of health locked away which needs only to be tapped, processed, and then sold; and that the medical industry has products which are directly responsible for increases in health. It is still commonly believed that increases in the quantity of the 'health supply' (drugs and implements) are bound to lead to corresponding increases in levels of health.

3.   *That medical science has produced a body of certain knowledge which can be applied to bodies as bodies rather than bodies as people.*[51]

4.   *That the best way to cure disease is to reduce bodies to their smallest constituent parts.* At the core of medical science there is the view that human bodies are nothing more than complicated biochemical machines. It is believed that there is an unbroken chain of cause and effect in physical disease which can best be attacked at its most fundamental level. The effect of this outlook is that molecular and electrochemical disturbances and abnormalities have become the main focus for medicine, while other influences on people are afforded less attention. It is also thought that this 'certain knowledge' can be applied impartially to all sets of molecules, without regard to the person or to the person's interaction with the world.

5.   *That health can be quantified in relation to norms for populations, particular groups of individuals, and individuals.*

6.   *That medicine is and should be a form of engineering.* It is assumed that a doctor can and should separate herself from her subject just as an engineer can when she works out how best to maintain a bridge. It is further assumed that the upkeep of health is a matter of technical proficiency – that the doctor merely needs to keep tissues and molecules in their correct order in order to ensure normal functioning.

Problems

Medical science undoubtedly helps people overcome a range of physical and mental difficulties. However, it is high time the discipline took proper heed of the many criticisms that are repeatedly made of it. For example:

1.   Both medical education and practice are predominantly concerned with the structure and function of the body, and with disease processes. Medicine is practised mainly in hospitals and clinics. Although medicine instigates 'public health' and epidemiological research, such investigations are almost always focused on diseases, usually with little if any attention to the wider social and economic causes. The sociological literature is full of studies and arguments that show that the best ways of dealing with disease and illness are not necessarily those which concentrate on curing biochemical abnormalities.[52]

2.   Medical science disregards people's unquantifiable aspects. It treats our instincts, emotions and spiritual being as mostly irrelevant to medical practice, and so demeans and disrespects us.

3.   Medical science typically assumes that full objectivity is possible – at least in the sense that doctors can be totally detached from their patients. However, work in the philosophy of science has shown that this degree of objectivity is impossible, and that medical scientists are not as removed from their subjects as some of them believe (see **Update** below for a more complete discussion of this point).

4.   The idea that health can be quantified can, according to some medical thinking, be translated into the definition that health is the normal state of individuals and populations. This emphasis on quantification has its advantages, since statistics and measurement can provide a sharp gauge for practical treatment and care. There are obviously a great many features of individuals and populations that can be measured. For example it is possible to measure: levels of haemoglobin; the average number of children per family; the major sources and amounts of protein in a population's diet; the height, mobility, and speech of a child at a certain age; life expectancy, and so on *ad infinitum*. These features can be surveyed and analysed in order to calculate a 'normal condition'. If this norm is not being achieved then steps may be taken to improve the situation.

However, what is worrying about this definition is that, taken on its own as the criterion of health, it can act to justify an existing state of affairs which would, on other standards, be described as undesirable. The definition implies that the normal standard – whatever this may be – is healthy. Yet the normal 'state of health' of children in a poverty-stricken village in South America and the normal 'state of health' of children in a prosperous California suburb differ drastically. Which children are healthy?

Work in the sociology of medicine heightens the worry. A common theme in this discipline is that health is often used as a normative term (i.e. as a term which *establishes* a norm by prescribing a standard – see comment in **Update**). And if health is defined according to prevailing social values (which is typically how norms are established) then it could be argued that both groups of children – those in South and North America – are healthy. It simply depends which norms one chooses to apply.

Consider these cases: the history of medicine records that the haemoglobin levels of young women in a Victorian workhouse were measured and an average calculated. This quantified norm was then assumed to be the correct standard of health, but this was a relatively poor standard. The haemoglobin levels of the women were so low that they suffered from chlorosis (a form of anaemia in which the skin takes on a greenish colouration), but since they had been defined as healthy their peculiar skin colour and lack of energy was explained as being a normal physiological condition of young women during puberty.[53]

This is the problem in a nutshell:

1.   Since claims about health are normative, it is possible to set varying standards of health.

2. If one decides to adopt relative standards then one may accept norms in some places and circumstances that are less than those in other places and circumstances – thus lowering expectations and fostering conservatism.

3. If one opts for universal standards instead, there are still problems:

    a. How does one choose what universal standard to adopt?
    b. How does one decide what to measure?
    c. The decision about what to measure and what not to measure is not value-free – if one chooses traditional medical criteria (as **WHO** mostly does) then *this* normative judgement places these understandings of health above other possible understandings of health.

IVAN ILLICH'S CASE AGAINST MEDICINE

The foremost critic of medicine in recent years is the theologian, and lifelong opponent of state systems, Ivan Illich. His criticisms of the medical establishment raise further questions about the medical approach.

Illich takes the view that modern medicine has created new types of disease. He writes:

> The medical establishment has become a major threat to health. The disabling impact of professional control over medicine has reached the proportions of an epidemic. (p. 11)[45]

Illich insists that for the most part medicine is itself a major impediment to the achievement of health. He discusses iatrogenesis, by which he means diseases, sufferings or obstacles actually created by medical intervention:

> Increasing and irreparable damage accompanies present industrial expansion in all sectors. In medicine this damage appears as iatrogenesis. Iatrogenesis is clinical when pain, sickness and death result from medical care; it is social when health policies reinforce an industrial organisation that generates ill-health; it is cultural and symbolic when medically sponsored behaviour and delusions restrict the vital autonomy of people by undermining their competence in growing up, caring for each other, and ageing, or when medical intervention cripples personal responses to pain, disability, impairment, anguish and death. (p. 271)[45]

Illich provides substantial lists of the 'harmful side effects' of many drugs and numerous accounts of 'unnecessary surgery'. He argues that surgery and chemo-therapy are actually new forms of epidemic and that scientific medicine has made all of us patients. We are now so subordinate to medicine that the essence of our humanity – our autonomy – is seriously threatened. Now that the more fatal epidemics have disappeared modern medicine has set about creating its own. According to Illich, medicine must do this in order to remain as an instrument for the bureaucratic control of human society.

Illich's polemic makes the most sense once one understands what he means by health. Illich thinks:

> Health designates a process of adaptation. It is not the result of instinct, but of an autonomous yet culturally shaped reaction to socially created reality. It designates the

ability to adapt to changing environments, to growing up and ageing, to healing when damaged, to suffering, and to the peaceful expectation of death. Health embraces the future as well, and therefore includes anguish and the inner resources to live with it... Health is a task, and as such is not comparable to the physiological balance of the beasts. Success in this personal task is in large part the result of self-awareness, self-discipline, and inner resources by which each person regulates his own daily rhythm and actions, his diet and his sexual activity. (pp. 273–274)[45]

Illich's point is that conscious, rather than merely biological, adaptation is an essential part of being a person. Health is a process of adaptation which is dependent on personal autonomy. For Illich autonomy itself is not health, but it is necessary for health (he says 'health [is the result of]...an autonomous yet culturally shaped reaction to socially created reality'). Autonomy cannot be entirely given since it depends in part on personal qualities and energies, but it can be prevented if a person is placed in a situation where, for instance, he cannot choose his response because through ignorance he is in no position to do so.

Illich considers the 'medicalisation of life' to be part of the general counter-productivity of an over-industrialised society (a theme he has explored in other contexts such as education and energy utilisation).[54] Because it involves a loss of autonomy, Illich believes that the harm caused by this counter-productivity is political. He argues that consequently a political solution is required. In the case of medicine this means that individuals must reassert personal control over their health: people must be allowed to adapt freely, which means that medical interference must be kept to a minimum.

Illich is emphatic that:

> Thoughtful public discussion of the iatrogenic pandemic, beginning with an insistence upon the demystification of all medical matters, will not be dangerous to the commonweal. Indeed what is dangerous is a passive public that has come to rely on superficial medical house-cleanings. The crisis in medicine could allow the layman effectively to reclaim his own control over medical perception, classification and decision making. The laicization of the Aesculapian temple could lead to the delegitimizing of the basic religious tenets of modern medicine to which industrial societies, from the left to the right, now subscribe...the layman and not the physician has the potential perspective and effective power to stop the current iatrogenic epidemic. (p. 12)[45]

Illich's optimistic position is that non-medically qualified people will somehow be able to convince the medics and the medical industry that the medical establishment will have to be dismantled. He explains that the present 'medical nemesis' is experienced by people who are 'largely deprived of any autonomous ability to cope with nature, neighbours, and dreams, and who are technically maintained within environmental, social and symbolic systems' – in other words people who have been conditioned to fit neatly into society's slots. Such 'lay-people' will have to acquire the knowledge and competence to evaluate the impact of medicine on health, and yet in reality it is only the medical establishment that could possibly make this happen.

Much of what Illich has to say makes sense. Certainly his remarks should be read by all consumers and providers of medicine, but such a noisy harangue can cover up gaps not filled by reasoned argument. His research into the various forms of iatrogenesis is extensive and impressive and has not been refuted, but what he says about medicine is too black and white. The following points in particular can be made against his position:

1.   There is not such a direct link between people lacking autonomy and the practice of medical science as Illich imagines. There are many social reasons why people are not autonomous and do not develop their potentials (and this has always been so, in all societies throughout history). Furthermore, medical science can enhance autonomy: medicine frequently relieves problems which would otherwise act against individual autonomy. Autonomy is affected if an individual has to spend his time caring for and trying cure himself of disease and illness, and if his problem limits the activities he would normally do.

Illich gives medical science little credit. Antibiotics can be used to control infection and are not always used unwisely. Pain relief has become sophisticated, and not all surgery is unnecessary. For instance hip-replacement operations and heart bypass surgery can be most enabling, and are now commonplace. In addition, the understanding of the causes of disease has undeniably increased.

2.   Is Illich's vision realistic? How can the changes he suggests be brought about? He does not tell us. In his discussion of the problems caused by medicine he does not cover the full reality of the situation. He does not propose a solution from 'where we are now', but from a point at which it would be conceivable for things to change quickly. There are countless factors that are bound to affect autonomy, such as traditions of behaviour, pollution, and corporate competition, which cannot be altered by individuals, however autonomous we are singly. In order to bring about the sweeping changes Illich recommends people must come together in groups – collective action is necessary, but to join a group inevitably means sacrificing some autonomy in order to achieve collective goals.

Illich gives little indication of the form his proposed 'self-care' should take. In one sense this is precisely his point – specifications and rule-following are anathema to independent thinking. However, he also says that people whose lives have been 'medicalised' are 'largely deprived of any autonomous ability to cope with nature, neighbours, and dreams, and are technically maintained within environmental, social and symbolic systems'. And if this is the case then reasoned personal strategies are needed to enable people to deal with their environments and social pressures. Most people, as they are in the real world now, need at least some guidelines in order to begin to gain the confidence to adapt autonomously.

At times Illich seems to be advocating a return to Dubos' mythical 'golden age'. Witness these quotes:

> Famine will increase until the trend towards capital-intensive food production by the poor for the rich has been replaced by a new kind of labour intensive, regional, rural autonomy. (p. 266)

> A world of optimal and widespread health is obviously a world of minimal and only occasional medical intervention. (p. 274)[45]

But this is not obvious at all.

3.   Although Illich argues that care should be done to oneself and occur within families he neglects the significant number of cases in which neither of these forms of care are possible. Young children, many elderly, the congenitally handicapped, the mentally ill, some accident victims, people with degenerative diseases (such as multiple sclerosis), the terminally ill, and others, are unable to care for themselves and often cannot be cared for within families. They may not have families, and if they do then the autonomy of the carer will almost inevitably become subservient to the maintenance of the sufferer – an unsatisfactory state of affairs on Illich's own account. For cases such as these there is a need for a system of welfare (which presumably would have to be bureaucratically organised and run by specially trained staff) which does not place a total burden on individuals and families already suffering severely. Admittedly this welfare system need not rest on medical foundations, but, given the existing state of affairs and the possible natures of the problems of the sufferers, it seems highly unlikely that medicine would be out of bounds.

In sum, Illich's main difficulty is that shared by all who advocate versions of the theory that health is an ability to adapt. He does not properly explain the nature of this ability, nor does he discuss how such an ability can be created and enhanced.

THE HUMANIST APPROACH

As noted earlier in this chapter, humanism is a label which can cover a range of theories, and there is no single doctrine which can fully demarcate it.[55]

It is better to think of humanism as an attitude – as a way of living and believing – based on a fairly fluid set of themes in humanist thought. For me, humanism is an outlook which holds that the common interests of individual human beings are of primary importance and should take preference over more particular interests. All policies, whether scientific, medical, social, political, industrial or some other should take full account of the abilities of human beings to make reasoned choices, and to work to develop ourselves.

Humanism is opposed to the belief that single solutions can be found which will apply universally to the ever-changing problems of human life. Humanism resists and counteracts dogmatism, and stands against the propagation of 'blind knowledge'. Humanism acknowledges that practical knowledge is necessary for many tasks but condemns in all cases the sort of 'education' which prefers training people to follow only given procedures rather than enabling them to think for themselves. Humanism challenges the view that people ought to follow policies which someone else has decided are in their best interests if the individuals concerned have not been given the information necessary for them to make their own judgements.

The most basic humanist position is that human dignity depends upon self-determination. This capacity for free choice is the source of morality: without the possibility of choice there is no possibility of morality. As a consequence, humanism does not lay down hard and fast specific moral rules. A humanist has faith in his fellow human beings, believing that with increased autonomy people will come to recognise and respect other people's potentials: the recognition of the fullness of one's own humanity will generate a heightened feeling for the humanity and common interests of others.

When stated in the abstract such dictums as 'do not do unto others what you would not wish for yourself', 'the rightness or wrongness of an action depends on the effect of that action on the welfare of all human beings', or 'act so that the effect of your action is compatible with the permanence of genuine human life' can appear to be nothing more than well-meaning platitudes, and certainly there are many instances where the practical application of such general guides is highly debatable. However, this does not detract from the overall worth of such ideals. It is a humanist theme that such maxims, once personally thought through, should be heeded whenever significant decisions have to be taken.

With respect to health, humanism offers the view that health is a personal goal which people should be free to strive for through their own efforts. Humanists are convinced that all human beings possess a latent ability to develop ourselves, so long as we have the actual or potential ability to understand the implications of our actions. Humanism never treats people as objects, as medical science sometimes has a tendency to do. Instead it is believed that people are incredibly complex physical, emotional, intellectual, and spiritual wholes (where 'spiritual' is used to mean having spiritual experiences of the world, not only religious ones).[56]

Problems

Many tomes have been written in praise of humanism, and there are humanist journals which try to apply humanist principles to practical problems.[36] But the changes in society needed to bring about the humanist notion of health are so great that the debate usually takes place on a 'worthy' yet theoretical plane. What is needed is generally agreed amongst humanists. We need mutual tolerance and respect, a tolerance of other people's beliefs and customs, an awareness that other people have needs which are similar to our own, and we need an environment where people can choose and are then able to develop themselves in accord with their choices. The problem is that it is far from clear how these goals are to be achieved, and so discussion frequently hovers around the issue of what is the fundamental need. Opinion varies as to whether this is more and better education for all, the removal of class divisions, the provision of full employment, the undermining of personal ego, de-industrialisation, de-bureaucratisation, the elimination of nationalism, or general increase in material prosperity, amongst many other candidates.

What is needed is more earthy controversy. What is needed is a full theory of health which takes account of all that is good in humanism, but which also puts forward concrete proposals. Inevitably these proposals will not be acceptable to everyone, but it is essential that they are aired in the arena of practice. If they are wrong, or too woolly, then they must be shown to be wrong or woolly.

NOTE: The Christian approach is not explored in this book because, with the obvious difference that humanism is not a religious doctrine, this approach shares many of humanism's prejudices.

THE COMMON FACTOR

A number of points have emerged or solidified in this chapter.

1. *Health does not have a single uncontroversial meaning.*
Health does not have a core meaning waiting to be discovered. There is no undisputed example of health. This is demonstrated by the fact that different theories of health – each plausible in its own way – regard health in different and sometimes conflicting modes.

2. *Health can be seen as a means or as an end.*
Health can be regarded as an end in itself. This end can be different dependent on age, ability, circumstance, and so on. Health can also be seen as a means – a state which must be achieved in order that further ends can also be achieved. In many cases the achievement of the means can be a significant end in itself.

Health can be described as either a means or an end, dependent upon the point of view of the person who is giving the description. For instance a medic could claim that by curing a specific disease in a person she has restored that person to health, but the patient may still have to spend time adjusting and convalescing – he might have lost a job or his friends through his disease. The patient may see the doctor's work as a beginning, as a means which will allow him to return to normal life eventually – a process which may require much more of the patient than just being free from disease.

It can be useful to know that these two ways of viewing health exist. It can be important to point out to a person that what he sees as an end (perhaps it is his own physical well-being) is actually also a means by which he can begin to move in other directions. Perhaps he might go on to attempt personal intellectual growth, or he might choose to help others achieve their own physical well-being.

3. *People cannot be fully understood in isolation from what they do in their lives. Also people cannot be fully understood in only biological terms.*
We have a great range of facets. Because of this diversity it is inevitable that specialist approaches designed to increase health will have different priorities and goals.

4. *Although there are some conflicts between the various theories and approaches there is an important common factor.*
This common factor is, on the face of it, blindingly simple. All the theories and approaches share an underlying sense, even though they take health to have different meanings. The common factor is that:

> *All theories of health and all approaches designed to increase health are intended to advise against, to prevent the creation of, or to remove, obstacles to the achievement of*

human potential. These obstacles may be biological, environmental, societal, familial, or personal.

This is why work for health is bound to be diverse. For example, in the cause of health a surgeon will operate to remove a tumour in order to give the organ or organs affected by the tumour's intrusion the chance to achieve the potential it or they would have if not restricted by the tumour – which can be thought of as a *liability*. Or a physician will prescribe antibiotics in order to allow the body to continue its development unimpaired by unbeneficial influences. Such work almost always enables people to fulfil other potentials in their lives.

Social workers, health visitors, and politicians work to remove different obstacles to the achievement of potential. For instance, they may try to eliminate problems such as lack of heating, damp conditions, marital trouble, child abuse, unemployment, or poor employment. Such impediments may cause further impediment such as disease and illness, and they act in their own right to divert time and energy from avenues along which to achieve more important potentials. In yet another way professional health educators advise against practices thought likely to create obstacles, and they may explain how a change in behaviour might help to remove existing obstacles.

All these activities are work for health.

The elimination or prevention of obstacles is by no means only a negative operation. Elimination and prevention of obstacles to potential does not only involve cutting away. The removal of impediment can often be achieved only through addition. Obstacles can be created by such disabling factors as ignorance, cultural deprivation, insufficiently developed powers of conceiving, apathy, lack of hope, lack of competence, and lack of confidence. Such impediments can be remedied only by positive measures of change and addition. For instance, it is important, in order to eliminate some obstacles, to provide more information and also more time to allow people to learn how to use and adapt this information to their own circumstances. And it is important to change environments, or social structures, or power possession, or prevailing attitudes and atmospheres, in order to provide more opportunity for people to begin to develop themselves. In other words, in order to remove many obstacles to achievement it is necessary to provide the right conditions for human flourishing.

It is now clear that issues of health are not only issues of disease and medicine. Health topics are inextricably linked with wider issues, issues about how people can and ought to conduct their lives. For many people it is the way in which a person is able to live that is the essential difference between health and ill health, regardless of bodily fortune or ill-luck. It is only for those convinced by mechanistic theories that health is a separate issue from personal life.

Katherine Mansfield knew this well. She wrote:

> By health I mean the power to live a full, adult, living, breathing life in close contact with what I love – the earth and the wonders thereof – the sea – the sun, all that we mean when we speak of the external world. I want to enter into it, to be part of it, to live in it, to

learn from it, to lose all that is superficial and acquired in me and to become a conscious, direct human being. I want, by understanding myself, to understand others. I want to be all that I am capable of becoming so that I may be . . . a child of the sun . . . But warm, eager, living life – to be rooted in life – to learn, to desire to know, to feel, to think, to act. That is what I want. And nothing less. That is what I must try for. (pp. 278–279)[44]

When extracted from her passionate prose, Mansfield's definition of health is *the power to achieve* or *the power to truly be*. Hers is a more poetic version of the more rigorous and analytic theory put forward in the next chapter.

AN OBJECTION

It is time the devil had an advocate.

> So far we have been led by the hand through several apparently plausible stages. We realise there is a real problem about stating clearly whether or not a person is healthy, and we know words can be used ambiguously. We see that there is a need to clear things up in the health field, and we recognise that there can be different theories of health, all of which have their problems. We are also prepared to accept that a common factor in health work is the removal of different obstacles to different human potentials. But now we are being manoeuvred into accepting the truth of a further position *that a person's state of health cannot realistically be separated from a person's quality of life*. We have reached a point where we are no longer being coaxed. We are being led by the nose. We wish to go no further.
>
> There are several protests we could make, but one basic objection may be enough to show that the argument has already gone too far: there has been too much playing with words – too many liberties have been taken. Most of the theories and approaches discussed stretch the meaning of the word health too far in order to suit their particular purposes, and the idea that good health is equivalent to a good quality of life has stretched meaning beyond breaking point.
>
> In reality health is a narrower topic than has been argued. Most of the theories of health, and most of the uses of the word health cited, are wrong. Health services are correctly named. Health services pay attention to diseases and illnesses for the single purpose of restoring people to health. Health is the speciality of health services. Other disciplines which claim to have an interest in health are merely tinkering. Health is a state which exists at one end of a continuum and has disease as its opposite, like this:
>
> HEALTH —————————— DISEASE
>
> Health and disease are personal states to be enjoyed or to be suffered. There are various states in between, in particular becoming ill and getting better.

RESPONSE

The objection is mistaken. Only in a limited sense do present Westernised health services work to restore health. This point cannot be made too often.

1. An inspection of any etymological dictionary will show that the meaning of a word is not fixed once and for all, and that one word can be used with several different meanings. The meanings of words do change, however there must always be limits, and it is important to clarify these.

A controversial contemporary example of how the meanings of words can evolve accompanies the present information technology revolution. Prior to the invention of electronic computers the word intelligence was correctly applied only to living organisms, and then almost exclusively to man and the higher mammals. Now that computers can perform complicated calculations at almost the speed of light, be programmed to design intricate blueprints, be programmed to program themselves, and be programmed to beat the best human chess players, it has become widely accepted that it is correct to talk of intelligent machines.

There are people who dislike and find serious fault with this practice, but they are in the minority, and their distaste for the new use of the word intelligent does not alter the fact that it is used meaningfully.

2.   There are alternatives to the medical model. These understandings of health have more in common with the idea of wholeness, which is the original meaning of health. These alternative views may complement and also conflict with the more limited medical view. Health can be thought of as an ability to fulfil a role, as a strength, and as an ability to adapt to changing circumstances. All the ideas share a common sense and each would form the basis of a broader health service than we have at present, were they to be put into practice.

3.   Even if health is thought to be the opposite of disease, even if this most limited meaning is chosen, then, because there are many and varied causes of disease and illness, wider factors than individual physiology and biochemistry must be taken into account. Social researchers such as Black, Mitchell, Acheson, and Doyal have produced a wealth of evidence which shows that such factors as living conditions, work, economic policies, stress, and different sorts of pollution can cause disease and illness.

4.   Present work within the health service is *already* wider than the idea of health put forward by the medical model. Many practising health educators and promoters, nurses, health visitors, counsellors, chaplains, and doctors try to help people perceived as wholes cope with life as a whole. They work to help with such problems as finance and benefits, with housing and home helps, with sorting out future options for people, and they also often look to help the close family and relatives of patients. All this is already done in the name of health.

5.   Health is not an absolute. Health is not a fixed state. The optimum states different people can achieve are inevitably different. Optimum states for single individuals are also different at different times in their lives. It is, therefore, mistaken to imagine health placed on a static continuum like the one presented above.

The idea that health is a specific, definable, fully describable state to which everyone can aspire equally is nonsense. It is as meaningless as the idea that there can be a perfect person. What would such a being be like?

THEORIES OF HEALTH – UPDATE

ADDITIONAL THEORIES OF HEALTH

Several more theories of health have emerged since – or were appearing around the time of – the publication of the first edition of *Health: the Foundations for Achievement.* These theories merit discussion, but none is sufficiently different to prompt a revision of the four categories of theory explained in this chapter.

THE SPECIES-TYPICAL THEORY OF HEALTH

This idea is that health is nothing more and nothing less than the opposite of disease. Its two most oft-cited proponents are Christopher Boorse and Norman Daniels. For Boorse disease is:

> ...the inability to perform all typical physiological functions with at least typical efficiency.[57]

The functions of a healthy organ are:

> ...its species typical causal contributions to the organism's survival and reproduction.[58]

Thus health is normal functioning, where normal means 'typical to the species design' and free of disease.[21]

Likewise for Daniels, who argues that in order to work for health a health care system should strive to remove barriers to normal opportunity due to disease, where 'disease' is understood as any 'adverse departure from normal species functioning'.

Problems with the Species-Typical Theory

The **species-typical theory of health** may be subsumed under **the theory that health is a commodity** and **the approach of medical science**, and its difficulties are mostly explained in the critiques of these two themes in this chapter: the conjunction of health with disease is not a *necessary* one, and although the statement 'health is what is normal for a species' may *look like* a neutral claim, the choice to associate health and disease is nevertheless a human judgement that what is statistically normal is good and what is not statistically normal is bad.

In addition, to select 'typical functioning' as the criterion for not being diseased (and so being healthy) leads to paradoxes that neither Boorse nor Daniels intend. For example, both want to say that viral and bacterial infections are diseases, and yet (particularly in winter) human beings typically suffer from them. Furthermore, the history of colonisation records numerous cases where the introduction of a previously unmet bacterium or virus wiped out the majority of a newly colonised population.[21,59] Following Columbus' and Cook's explorations, and the subsequent invasion of native territories by Europeans, about 90% of both native American and Polynesian populations died after exposure to infections (such as influenza) commonplace to the colonisers. The problem for both Boorse and Daniels is to explain how the species-typical reaction in these cases (i.e. to succumb to disease) can possibly be the healthy one. In the case of HIV infection in the present day, our species-typical reaction is to contract AIDS, yet a small number of *species-atypical* people seem to be able to resist the virus (how they do so is currently the subject of intense scientific research[60]) – but in this case (according to Boorse's and Daniels' 'commonsense' assumptions) it must again be the non-typical members who are healthy.

THE VITAL GOALS THEORY OF HEALTH

The Swedish philosopher Lennart Nordenfelt has advanced (independently) a fairly complex theory of health which has features in common with the **foundations theory**, but which is ultimately prescriptive (i.e. the upshot of Nordenfelt's theory is that it can be work for health to tell people what is best for them).

Nordenfelt claims that someone is healthy if she has the ability to reach her 'vital goals'. He defines 'vital goals' like this:

> x is a vital goal to P iff x is a state which is necessary for P's minimal happiness...[61]

In other words, a person will be healthy (at least to some degree) if she has the ability to achieve goals necessary to a basic level of happiness.

Problems with the Vital Goals Theory

Like the **foundations theory**, the (welcome) implication of the **vital goals theory** is that it is not only problems of disease and illness that can prevent health; all sorts of factors can affect a person's ability to achieve happiness. Crucially however, Nordenfelt's notion of health has to specify what the vital goals are, whereas the **foundations theory** holds that work for health is work to provide the wherewithal to enable people to decide for themselves how best to live. Consequently Nordenfelt is forced to say that vital goals are what is good for people (partly because he developed his theory as a result of an earlier interest in the philosophy of action, which is preoccupied with goal-directed behaviour), and that sometimes people do not know what is good for them. One of Nordenfelt's students, Per-Anders Tengland, explains:

> (For Nordenfelt) [W]hat a person *says* are her vital goals and what her vital goals *are* do not have to coincide. The individual can be mistaken.[62]

So a sadist or a paedophile, for example, may think their vital goals are to hurt others or to have sex with children, but these are not (for Nordenfelt) healthy things to do and so cannot be their true vital goals. However, while one might agree that these behaviours are undesirable, to say that they cannot count as actions towards 'vital goals' (and so toward health) if they do indeed make the perpetrators happy, is simply puritanism: Nordenfelt does not approve of what some other people call 'vital goals' and so they cannot be 'vital goals'. And the practical effect of this is that it becomes acceptable for health workers to impose their values on other people (a form of 'good life health promotion' I criticise in a later publication, *Health Promotion: Philosophy, Practice and Prejudice*[14]). Also see the discussion of 'health gain' in *Health Promotion* for a fuller account of the fundamental difference between Nordenfelt's theory and the **foundations theory**.

THE MAORI UNDERSTANDING OF HEALTH

Until the mid-1980s the Maori view of health was implicit in Maori culture. However, in response to the obvious fact that the New Zealand health system is based on Western philosophies and practices, Maori writers began to articulate a Maori theory of health (several different writers gave different – though basically harmonious – versions of it).[63]

It is generally agreed that the Maori understanding of health incorporates:

    i.   **Te Taha Wairua**
   ii.   **Te Taha Hinengaro**
  iii.   **Te Taha Tinana**
  iv.   **Te Taha Whanau**

i. Te Taha Wairua: Spiritual Wellbeing
Te Taha Wairua is that non-material spiritual 'vital essence' part of a person. It is the life force that determines who you are, what you are, where you come from, where you are going to and provides the vital link with ancestors who are perceived as omnipresent. Spiritual wellbeing is extremely important for Maori people and is acknowledged in their everyday lives by observing certain practices and procedures. The *tangihanga*, funeral ceremony is one of the most important events in Maori life. The deceased is often referred to as *taonga* (treasure). It is not only seen as an occasion to farewell the deceased and to share the loss with the bereaved family but one to ensure the safe, untroubled journey of the wairua (spirit) to the spirit world and the happy reconciliation of the family into the living world.

It is a difficult concept to explain as each person has his/her own idea of spirituality, knowing what it means for him/herself and how it can influence his/her way of life.

ii. Te Taha Hinengaro: Mental Wellbeing
Te Taha Hinengaro is the mental and emotional dimensions of a person. It recognises that the mind, thoughts and feelings cannot be separated from the body or the soul and that together they determine how people feel about themselves and thus their state of health. Self-esteem and self-confidence are important ingredients for good health.

iii. Te Taha Tinana: Physical Wellbeing
Te Taha Tinana is that dimension which recognises the physical or bodily aspect of a person. It is the part of a person that western medicine focuses upon. Maori people like many other groups believe that the mind, body and soul are all closely inter-related and influence the physical state of wellbeing. Physical health cannot be dealt with in isolation nor can the individual person be seen as separate from the family.

iv. Te Taha Whanau: Family Wellbeing

Te Taha Whanau acknowledges the importance of the function and role of the family in providing sustenance, support and an environment conducive to good health. There are many definitions of family. Maori people define it to include the extended family network that embraces all vertical and horizontal kinship members of a whanau, hapu or tribal group. *Whanaungatanga* (family relationships) is the essential element that provides a sense of belonging, identification and collective strength.[64]

The most popular expression of the above has been put forward by Mason Durie, a Maori academic. He writes:

> *Te Whare Tapa Wha*
> In 1983 Durie introduced the proposition that Maori views on health emphasised aspects different to [sic] conservative Western views. His... model compares health to the four walls of a meeting house – *te whare tapa wha*. Although each wall might be examined separately, all sides of the house are equally necessary to maintain strength, ensure shelter and give coherence... Each wall was seen to represent a different aspect of health: *te taha wairua*, a spiritual component, *te taha hinengaro*, a psychic component, *te taha tinana*, a bodily component, and *te taha whanau*, a family component.[65]

Problems with the Maori Theory

Like the **foundations theory**, the Maori understanding of health is holistic and includes much more than disease and illness in any assessment of a person's health. Furthermore, it explicitly incorporates *appreciation of community* (meaning at least extended family and deceased ancestors) as a part of what it is to be healthy.

Though I developed the **foundations theory of health** in complete ignorance of Maori culture, the similarities are striking (see **Figures 3 and 4**).

However, Western colonial influence is so insidious that even the most enlightened and culturally aware Maori thinkers sometimes vacillate between a holistic conception of health, and the alternatives shown in **Figures 1 and 2**.

For example:

> Efforts to encourage young Maori pre-schoolers to speak Maori stem to a large extent from a conviction that ill-health, be it in mental or physical spheres, is related to a loss of cultural skills and in particular an inability to communicate appropriately within a Maori context.[65]

and

> A second implication is that the biological substrate is only one indicator of health. The others include spiritual, psychological, interpersonal, family, economic and environmental dimensions. Policies that impinge on any one of those will impact on Maori health. In support of this point it may be noted that Barwick[66] has collated New Zealand evidence which shows that unemployment, low incomes and inadequate housing, for example, are major determinants of poor health.[65]

Close reading of these two excerpts from Durie's paper show just how powerful the Western understanding is. Remember that this is a Maori leader specifically writing to contrast the Maori view of health with the Western idea, yet even so there is *direct and*

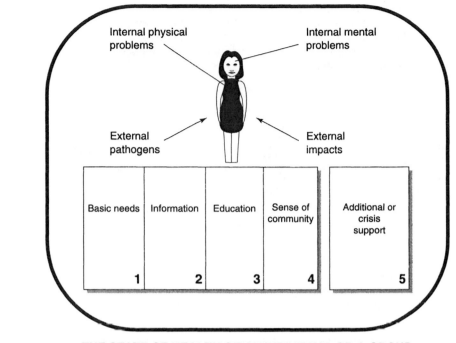

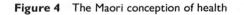

Figure 3   The foundations conception of health

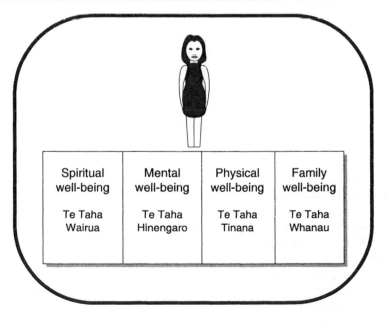

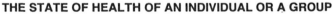

Figure 4   The Maori conception of health

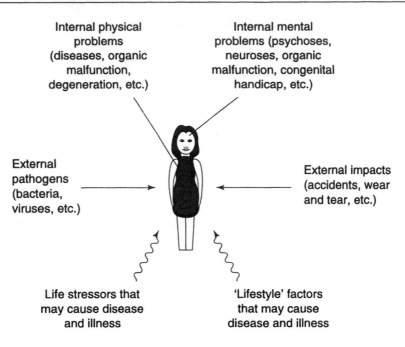

Internal physical
problems
(diseases, organic
malfunction,
degeneration, etc.)

Internal mental
problems (psychoses,
neuroses, organic
malfunction, congenital
handicap, etc.)

External
pathogens
(bacteria,
viruses, etc.)

External impacts
(accidents, wear
and tear, etc.)

Life stressors that
may cause disease
and illness

'Lifestyle' factors
that may cause
disease and illness

AN INDIVIDUAL WITH A HEALTH PROBLEM

Figure I   The conventional conception of health

repeated reference to health on the Western conception rather than the Maori one. Durie reports:

1.   'ill-health, be it in mental or physical spheres, is related to a loss of cultural skills'

and

2.   'unemployment, low incomes and inadequate housing, for example, are major determinants of poor health'.

However, in the first case, if he were to be true to the Maori understanding, he should have said 'loss of cultural skills *is* loss of health' (he used **conception two** when he should have used **conception four**). In the second case he cites evidence that people tend to have worse **health as the opposite of disease** the worse their living conditions (the Western view, an amalgam of **conceptions one** and **two**). But, to be consistent with the Maori view he himself advances, he should have referred to *'Te Whare Tapa Wha'*, according to which it is quite conceivable that health could increase as social conditions decrease (as, for example, a sense of *te taha wairua* and *te taha whanau* grows in response to adverse material conditions).

These theoretical errors – which simply must be avoided if Maori culture is ever to recover its pre-colonisation status – occur for the same reasons they occur in Anglo-Saxon theories of health – the theory has not been sufficiently explored and developed

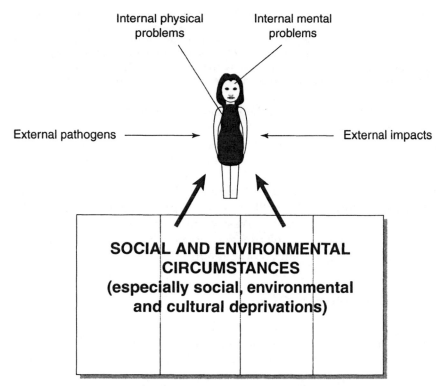

Figure 2   The socially aware conception of health

(and it deserves to be, not least because more Maori and other New Zealanders will understand it more clearly if it is).

CAROLINE WHITBECK'S THEORY OF HEALTH

Caroline Whitbeck's theory of health anticipated the **foundations theory**.[67] I must have read her paper as I was writing the first edition, though I cannot remember doing so. However, I assume it made a positive impression and probably helped me knock my own embryonic ideas into shape.

Summing up her theory she says:

> ... to say something is healthy or that it promotes health is to give a reason for saying that it is good. In contrast, the term 'disease' is value-laden in a distinct and hitherto unrecognised sense, that is, when we apply it to a psychophysiological process, we judge that the process is one that would be good (for people) to *be able* to prevent or treat effectively. The concepts of health and disease are not complementary concepts, therefore, but turn out to be concepts of different orders...

> Although it is important to understand the integrated character of a high state of health, significant components of health can be identified. Among these are physical fitness, having a realistic view of oneself and others, and having the ability to handle stressful situations. Although the concept of health is much more than the absence of disease, and indeed a high level of health is compatible with having some disease, health contrasts both with other aspects of social well-being and with happiness. (pp. 624–625)

Much of the basis of the **foundations theory** can be recognised in this brief quotation. For Whitbeck, as for myself, considerations of health are separate from matters of disease and illness, good health depends on a range of enabling factors integrating well with each other, being healthy is essentially to do with having abilities (or autonomy, in my favoured terminology), and health work neither encompasses all aspects of social support nor requires happiness. Both Whitbeck's theory and the **foundations theory** allow the possibility of an unhappy person being in good health (so sharing at least this aspect of the Western medical view), appreciating that to equate health with happiness (like Nordenfelt and establishment health promotion) is to take the first steps along an authoritarian path.

Problems with Whitbeck's Theory

The chief problem with Whitbeck's writing is that it really only hints at a theory. It is a pleasure to read, and is written with philosophical insight considerably in advance of most other contributions to the 'what is health?' debate, yet Whitbeck does not spell out the implications of her thinking, and so cannot hope to influence practice. Of course she may not have intended to make a practical difference, but by not testing the idea out in general life circumstances she misses a golden opportunity to develop a practical philosophy of health.

Whitbeck might also be criticised for incorporating her prejudice – for the primacy of individuals' rights – into her theory. But then she does so openly, clearly acknowledging that 'health is value-laden', and this in my view is infinitely to be preferred over more conventional assertions about health that disingenuously claim objectivity.

HOW THE FOUR THEORIES OF HEALTH RELATE TO THE THREE CONCEPTIONS

For the sake of further clarity, it is helpful to show how the four main **categories of theory of health** (see chart on p. 40) fit with the three different **conceptions of health** outlined in the introduction to the second edition.

---

1. **The theory that health is an ideal state**
    – A goal of perfect well-being in every respect.
    – An end in itself.
    – Disease, illness, handicap, and social problems must be absent.

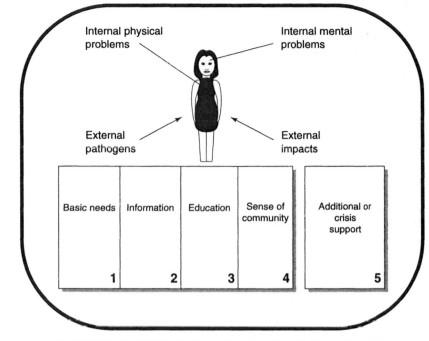

THE STATE OF HEALTH OF AN INDIVIDUAL OR A GROUP

Figure 3   The foundations conception of health

In principle – taken at its word – this theory of health is in keeping with the **foundations conception of health** as shown in **Figure 3**.

But the reality is rather different. **WHO** has developed and promoted this shining view of health for over half a century, capturing the imagination of countless health promoters who empathise with the idea that health is much more than 'the absence of disease or infirmity'. However, what **WHO** actually says and does is plainly medically inspired, so much so that one sincerely hopes there has been no duplicity in this regard. For example, the **WHO** website at: http://www.who.int/home/map_ht.html has this:

Governance | Health Topics | Information Sources | Reports | Site Map

HEALTH TOPICS

Diseases: communicable/infectious diseases
Diseases: tropical diseases
Diseases: vaccine preventable diseases
Environment
Family and reproductive health
Health policies, statistics, and systems
Health technology
Lifestyle
Non-communicable diseases

Diseases: Communicable/Infectious Diseases

Disease Outbreak News
Blindness and deafness
Bovine spongiform encephalopathies (BSE)
Buruli Ulcer
Cholera
Dysentery
Ebola haemorrhagic fever
Haemorrhagic fevers
Hepatitis
HIV/AIDS
Influenza
Leprosy
Meningitis
Plague
Rabies
Sexually transmitted diseases
Tuberculosis
Zoonoses

Diseases: Tropical Diseases

African trypanosomiasis (sleeping sickness)
Chagas disease (American trypanosomiasis)
Dengue
Dracunculiasis
Leishmaniasis (kala azar)
Lymphatic filariasis
Malaria
Onchocerciasis (river blindness)
Schistosomiasis (bilharzia)

Diseases: Vaccine Preventable Diseases

Acute respiratory virus
Diphtheria
Dengue
Haemophilus influenzae
Hepatitis B
Japanese encephalitis
Measles
Meningococcal
Mumps
Neonatal tetanus
Pertussis
Poliomyelitis
Rotavirus
Pneumococcal
Shigella
Tuberculosis
Typhoid fever
Varicella
Vitamin A deficiency
Yellow fever

Non-Communicable Diseases

Asthma
Cancer
Cardiovascular diseases
Chronic rheumatic diseases
Diabetes
Human genetic-related diseases
Non-communicable diseases
Noma
Oral Health
Tobacco Use
World No-Tobacco Day

Environment

Air
Chemical safety
Climate and Health
Drinking Water Quality
Electromagnetic fields (EMF)
Environmental epidemiology
Environmental health
Environmental sanitation
Food Safety
Health, environment and development
Healthy cities
Noise
Occupational health
Radiation safety
Rehabilitation
Solar UV Radiation
Solid and Hazardous Wastes
Water supply and sanitation
WHO Pesticide Evaluation Scheme (WHOPES)
Women, health and environment

Family and Reproductive Health

Acute respiratory infections
Adolescent health and development
Children's vaccination
Cholera
Diarrhoeal disease
Immunization
Integrated management of childhood illness
Reproductive health
Reproductive health research
Reproductive tract infections
Women's health

Health Policies, Statistics, and Systems

Biotechnology
Country cooperation
Drugs and medicines
Drug safety

Emergency and humanitarian action
Epidemiological Information
Essential drugs
Health policy
Health statistics
Health technology
Statistical information
Support to countries in greatest need

It is surely unreasonable to trumpet health as:

...a state of complete physical, mental and social well-being and not merely the absence of disease and infirmity

when virtually all **WHO**'s 'health topics' actually concern disease and infirmity. This is not to say that it is not important to try to combat disease – indeed this is one of the things we are biologically programmed to do[68] – but it is to say that it is quite wrong to secure the massive funding necessary to do so under such a misleading slogan. If only a small proportion of **WHO**'s government grants were to be redirected to non-medical health projects (like restoring colonised people's sense of culture or on development projects for mental health not controlled by psychiatry, for example) then the foundational health gains would be immense.

At one website[69] **WHO** makes this claim for its Healthy Cities programme:

The Healthy Cities Program makes this proposition: 'with the help of our partners in local government together we could engage the broader community in a grand endeavor – a global mission to transform the living and health conditions of people, in every country.'

In so doing (and simply through habit) it makes a distinction between 'the living and health conditions of people', so slipping – as it does so often – into **conceptions one** or **two**.

If **WHO** was true to its definition it could not distinguish between conditions of life (i.e. general living conditions) and conditions of health (for **WHO**, those factors that are or might become the subject of clinical work), but of course it does so time and time again because **WHO**'s stated definition of health is not its real one.

At another website[70] and within the two opening sentences, **WHO** explicitly correlates mental health with mental illness, when this is not a necessary relationship. **WHO** clearly sees more psychiatry as the way to improve mental health, and this is not a necessary relationship either.[71]

Mental health problems are dramatically increasing. Data suggest that mental health problems are among the most important contributors to the global burden of disease and disability. Neuropsychiatric disorders measured by DALYs represent 11.5% of the global burden of disease. Among the neuropsychiatric disorders unipolar depression alone accounts for 36.5% (10.4% bipolar depression, 11.3% alcohol dependence, 8.7% psychosis, 3.5% epilepsy). According to 1990 estimates, 5 of the 10 leading causes of disability are mental disorders: unipolar major depression, alcohol dependence, bipolar depression, schizophrenia and obsessive–compulsive disorder. Beyond the striking figures related to those suffering from defined mental disorders, there exist a number of groups of people who because of extremely difficult conditions or circumstances are at special risk of being affected by the burden of mental health problems. These include children and adolescents experiencing disrupted nurturing, abandoned elderly, abused women, those traumatized by war and violence, refugees and displaced persons, many indigenous people and obviously persons in extreme poverty. To respond to such a dramatic challenge the World Health Organization is substantially expanding its investment in mental health and the Department of Mental Health and Substance Dependence represents one of its major arms for this purpose.

Note the first sentence in particular – apparently the trouble with health problems is that they increase 'the global burden of disease and disability' – yet according to **WHO**'s Constitution this global health burden is 'merely' a matter of disease and infirmity, by no means the whole story of health. So – one might be forgiven for asking **WHO** – where is the rest of the story, and how are you spending our money to improve it?

In sum, sometimes **WHO** uses **conception two** and at other times **conception one** – but never **conception three**, just because of its unprovable and territorial assumption that health is the opposite of disease and so the primary concern of medicine and associated disciplines.

---

2. The theory that health is the physical and mental fitness to do socialised daily tasks (i.e. to function normally in a person's own society)
 – A means toward the end of normal social functioning.
 – All disease, illness and handicap which disable normal functioning must
   be absent.
 – Chronic illnesses, diseases and handicaps can be present.

This category clearly coincides with **conception one** (see **Figure 1**).

The individual is the focus and may – though need not automatically – fall into the 'sick role' as he contracts disease, illness and injury.

---

3. The theory that health is a commodity that can be bought or given
 – The rationale which underlies medical practice.
 – Usually perceived as an end for the provider, a means for the receiver.
 – The more disease, illness, pain and injury, the poorer the health of the patient.
 – Health may be restored piecemeal, through therapies offered by
   distinct specialisms.

This category also coincides most typically with **conception one**.

---

4. A group of theories which hold that health is a personal strength or ability – either physical, metaphysical or intellectual
 – These strengths and abilities are not commodities, and cannot normally be
   given or purchased. They may exist innately, or they may be developed
   by individuals on their own, by individuals working together, or by
   individuals receiving support from others. These strengths and abilities
   can also be lost.

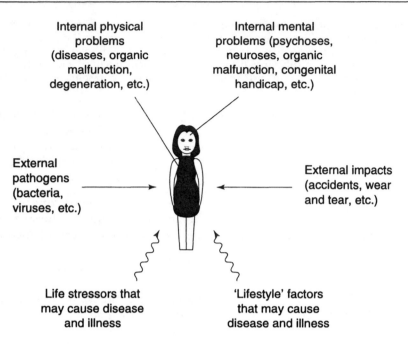

Internal physical
problems
(diseases, organic
malfunction,
degeneration, etc.)

Internal mental
problems (psychoses,
neuroses, organic
malfunction, congenital
handicap, etc.)

External
pathogens
(bacteria,
viruses, etc.)

External impacts
(accidents, wear
and tear, etc.)

Life stressors that
may cause disease
and illness

'Lifestyle' factors
that may cause
disease and illness

AN INDIVIDUAL WITH A HEALTH PROBLEM

Figure I   The conventional conception of health

This category has most in common with **conceptions three and two**. However, it is not sufficiently clearly expressed by its advocates to enable a more precise designation.

CHAPTER FIVE

The Fullest Sense of Health

REVIEW

What ground has been covered so far in this philosophical exploration? What progress have we made?

Looking back over the previous chapters, it has become apparent that there is no simple answer to the question 'What is health?' The idea that health is desirable, that it is a 'good thing' to have, and that this is all that can really be said on the subject is clearly not good enough. Different people have different ideas about health, and therefore inevitably disagree about whether Dennis and the other case studies are healthy or not. People from different backgrounds, with different sets and orderings of values can, quite plausibly, mean different things when they speak of health. And this is frustrating – we naturally expect commonly used words to have clear definitions.

The question 'How to be clear about the meaning of health?' was left in the air briefly, while a general problem about the meaning of our most important words was explained in **Chapter Three**. The problem is by no means exclusive to the word 'health', in fact it affects the majority of human communications for the worse. We must recognise it, and we must continually attempt to deal with it. And the way to do this is through philosophy – a process of clarification that digs to the taproots of problems:

> Philosophical problems are not empirical problems; they are solved rather by looking into the workings of our language, and that in such a way as to make us recognise those workings: in despite of an urge to misunderstand them. The problems are solved, not by giving new information, but by arranging what we have always known. Philosophy is a battle against the bewitchment of our intelligence by means of our language.[72]

Various theories about health were assessed in **Chapter Four**. Each tries to answer the question 'What is health?' differently. None of them is fully compatible with any other, and so they cannot be combined into a comprehensive theory of health, and each creates further puzzles. For example, precisely what is ideal health? How can such a target be specified? How can health be equivalent to being able to fulfil a social role if that role is making a person depressed? If health is strength how can we work to create this strength? Is bowing to fate the most we can do? How can we define the difference between positive and negative adaptation to changing circumstances? Dying after being run over by a bus is a form of adaptation – so is suicide, so is wife-beating, so is alcoholism, and so is safe-breaking. Arguably all these practices are debilitating. How can such strength-sapping reactions be distinguished from life-enhancing adaptations?

What is the next step? Can we abandon the problem here? Should we accept that health is an idea that is forever contestable? Can we leave it that the limits of its meaning can ebb, flow, and bend at the whim of any new theorist, however crazy or clever, who claims to have discovered what health is really about?

We have discovered that all theories about health and all approaches designed to improve it share at least one element in common. They each ascribe different meanings to the word 'health' but agree, implicitly at least, that work for health is work towards the removal of obstacles which face people daily. This is progress. Is it possible to go further? An effort must be made because we all face so many obstacles to our ambitions, and not every obstacle can be the concern of health workers. We have not yet gone far enough in explaining the nature of health. We need to probe deeper still. The fact that I would like my car sprayed a different colour but cannot afford it because I did not sell enough copies of the first edition of this book is an obstacle to me, but even I cannot argue that this obstacle should be the direct concern of my local health workers.

WHAT MORE IS NEEDED IN ORDER TO OFFER AN ADEQUATE THEORY OF HEALTH?

A comprehensive and useful theory of health should avoid the pitfalls encountered by the theories described in the previous chapters. A full theory of health must also:

1. *Propose a limit both to health's meaning and to practical work for health.*
The theory must propose a limit to the legitimate meanings of health, and must do so as clearly as possible. The theory must be able to acknowledge the breadth of the possible uses of the word health, but it must also be able to explain that work for health is not totally inclusive. Not all aspects of human life are to do with work for health.

2. *Acknowledge disagreement.*
The theory must recognise that people can disagree about the nature of health and yet each be partially correct. The theory needs to recognise that the conflicts between other theories and approaches cannot be resolved simply by saying theory X is wrong, theory Y is wrong, theory Z is correct, and so on. The issue is not as simple as this.

The theory must be able to throw calm on these troubled waters. It must be able to put the conflicts into perspective.   The theory must be able to show that although there are real disagreements, these need not cause head-on collisions. For instance, an adequate theory of health must be able to show that medical theories of health are not bound to confront theories which hold that health is essentially the ability to adapt to life's problems. Although the theories are set against each other at some levels, the conflicts are not as deep as the implicit agreement about the fundamental goal of health work.

3. *Be useful.*

An adequate theory of health must be a useful theory. There is little point, other than for intrinsic interest, in abstract debate for its own sake. The theory must be applicable by policy-makers, administrators, health educators, medics, nurses, teachers, and neighbours. Indeed the theory must be applicable by everyone who seeks health, either on their own behalf or on the behalf of others (See the Practical Applications of the Foundations Theory of Health in **The Fullest Sense of Health – Update**, below).

4. *Articulate the idea of degrees of health.*

Because it is a mistake to think of health as an absolute, an adequate theory must be able to articulate the idea that there can be degrees of health. Health assessment does not boil down to a choice of either/or – either Dennis is healthy or not. Without this deeper understanding the case of real Dennises will forever remain in black and white dispute, with the possible consequence that the help they are given, or can give themselves, will not be clear or will be too restricted.

5. *Be measurable.*

An adequate theory of health must allow measurement. In order to judge the effectiveness of work for health it must be possible to evaluate people's health, even when health is thought of in the fullest, holistic sense. Without this it will be impossible to reach shared conclusions about the impact of work for health.

6. *Be realistic.*

The theory must not appear unrealistic. It should not be out of step with current usage (for this would mean that it would be out of step with the other theories of health too, and would not share the common factor). It must still remain correct to write slogans such as:

> Cigarettes can seriously damage your health.

It must still be correct to say 'I have good health' and to mean only that one is in good physical condition. An adequate theory of health should aim to change not by confronting people, not by saying 'you have been wrong all these years', but by enriching personal concepts of health, by providing people with developed ideas which make sense of work they are doing already. New theories must filter gently into consciousness in order to be accepted.

This is a tall order. However the **foundations theory of health** proposed in this chapter is up to the challenge. To help show how, it is worth considering an idea Socrates put forward, and a diagram which tries to put words into pictures.

SOCRATES' THOUGHTS ON ROUNDNESS

As we saw earlier with the example of justice, Socrates was intrigued by 'what is?' questions. He appreciated that nothing is as simple as it first appears, and that the task of defining does not escape this maxim. Socrates did not attempt to define 'health', as far as we know, but his inquiries into the meaning of other words are enlightening. For example, Socrates tried to define 'roundness', asking: What does 'being round' mean?

We describe many objects as round even though they are not exactly the same. So it makes sense to ask: What are the limits beyond which we would not wish to describe objects as round? Socrates' proposals about this are complicated and involve what is known as The Theory of Forms.[19] Socrates thought that (somewhere) there exists a perfect and unchanging example of roundness – a standard against which all actual examples of roundness in the real world can be only imperfect copies. All actual examples imitate the perfect form to a recognisable degree.

This aspect of Socrates' argument is not important here. It is not helpful, and too similar to the inadequate **WHO** definition, to suggest that there is a perfect essence of health existing eternally, while all actual instances of health in this world are imitations of this perfection. Rather, the reason for introducing one of Socrates' central ideas – albeit in an oversimplified manner – is to point out that *to provide a satisfactory account of something it is not necessary to provide a precise definition. The essential task is to delimit – to show limits beyond which the account becomes unsatisfactory.*

Consider 'roundness': apples, oranges, rubber balls, cricket balls, and planets are all recognisably round. Tables (including their legs), squares and wooden poles are not round – these examples clearly exceed the limit of roundness. In the real world, this limit will always be fuzzy at the edges. For instance, is a plum round? Is an apple with a bite taken out of it round? In practice there will always be a certain fuzziness.

There will remain room for conflict and difference within the limit. The functions of apples, balls and planets are different. So too are their colours and sizes and textures. However, they all share the common feature 'roundness'.

It ought now to be easier to understand the point of saying that there is a limit to the sense of health that can be displayed fairly clearly, even though within this limit there can be real differences which cannot be, and do not have to be, resolved.

Socrates' idea about the limits to the meaning of 'roundness' can be illustrated by **Figure 5**.

HEALTH IS FOUNDATIONS FOR ACHIEVEMENT

Work for health is essentially *enabling*. It is a question of providing the appropriate foundations to enable the achievement of personal and group potentials. Health in its different degrees is created by removing obstacles and by providing the basic means by which biological and chosen goals can be achieved.

A person's (optimum) state of health is equivalent to the state of the set of conditions which fulfil or enable a person to work to fulfil his or her realistic chosen and biological potentials. Some of these conditions are of the highest importance for all people. Others are variable dependent upon individual abilities and circumstances.

The actual degree of health that a person has at a particular time depends upon the degree to which these conditions are realised in practice.

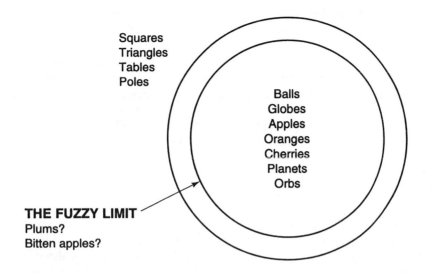

Figure 5   Socrates' thoughts on roundness. The Fuzzy limit

CENTRAL CONDITIONS

Some of the foundations which make up health are of the highest importance for all people. These are:

1.   *The basic needs of food, drink, shelter, warmth, and purpose in life (including spirituality and meaningfulness).*

2.   *Access to the widest possible information about all factors which have an influence on a person's life.*

3.   *The skill and confidence to assimilate this information.*
In most societies literacy and numeracy are needed in older children and adults. People need to be able to understand how the information applies to them, and to be able to make reasoned decisions about what action to take in the light of their information.

4.   *The recognition that an individual is never totally isolated from other people and the external world.*
People are complex wholes who cannot be fully understood separated from the influence of their environment, which is itself a whole of which they are a part. People are not like marbles packed in boxes, where they are a community only because of their forced proximity. People are part of their whole surroundings, like cells in a single body (I thank Dr Michael Wilson for these metaphors). This fact compels the recognition that a person should not strive to fulfil personal potentials which will undermine the basic foundations for achievement of other people. In short, an essential condition for health in human beings who are aware of the implications of their actions

is that they have an awareness of a basic duty they have because they are people in a community.

Other foundations for achievement are bound to vary between individuals dependent upon which potentials can realistically be achieved. For instance, a diseased person, a person in a damp and dilapidated house, a person in prison, a fit young athlete, a terminal patient, and an expectant mother all need the central conditions which constitute part of their healths, but in addition they require other specific foundations in order to enable them to make the most of their lives.

INFLUENCES ON HEALTH

As a small supplement to the vast literature on the range of factors which can cause disease and illness, a project was devised to inquire into the ways in which different groups of health care professionals think of health.[73] The first stage of the project was to concentrate on the nurses' concepts, and on how these might change during their training. Trainee nurses, qualified nurses, nurse tutors, health visitors, and district nurses were all asked what they think health is. Not unexpectedly the majority of the responses were vague. The **WHO** definition was sometimes cited, although it was usually described as 'not right'. If pressed, many of the interviewees put forward positions which quickly became contradictory.

A different line of attack was tried. The subjects were asked to 'List as many factors as you can which have a bearing on people's health'. The responses were surprisingly diverse. They included such factors as finance, food/diet, housing/warmth, electricity and gas boards (!), well-woman clinics, environment, family planning associations, smoking, transport, occupations, street lighting, culture, membership of ethnic groups, family pets, the National Health Service, private hospital care, sanitation, sewage, climate, safety factors, home accidents and factory accidents, restaurants, dairies, butchers, sexual relationships, jogging, lack of exercise, sedentary jobs, general practitioners, clothing, anxiety, stress, family pressures, education, unemployment, shopping areas, heredity, political decisions, social class, intelligence, crop spraying, other pollution, age, gender, religion, greed, fear, chiropody, government policy, prophylaxis, and the media.

It is clearly much easier to say what affects health than to say what health is. However, the research seems to show that practising health workers think about health in a way that is wider than disease cure and prevention. The **foundations theory** articulates these intuitions – all the above factors are legitimate influences on health according to it. The most commonly identified, and the most important, influences on health are those shown in **Figure 6**.

There are two main ways such influences can affect health (i.e. affect the strength of personal foundations):

1.   If they are bad, the influences can create obstacles in their own right. For example, lack of general education, having a black skin, experiencing poor living conditions, or having trouble in forming personal relationships, can lower the chances of a person

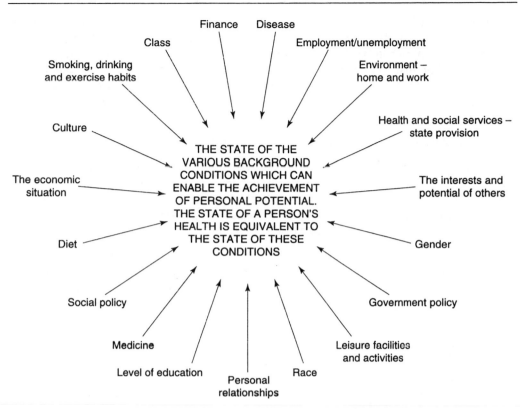

Figure 6   Influences on health

achieving a good range and level of his or her chosen and positive biological potentials.

2.   Such influences can create further obstacles of a kind more traditionally associated with health troubles. For example, it is now well known that a person's class and lifestyle can affect the probability of him becoming ill and diseased, that the type of work a person does can make it more or less likely that she will suffer from injury or stress, that smoking can cause disease and that the permitting of advertising and sports sponsorship by the tobacco companies persuades people to smoke, that poor personal relationships can cause depression and stress, and that lack of education about the way in which the body works can lead to injury.

All meaningful approaches to the creation of health – whether overtly political, medical, pastoral, or initiated by health visitors and social workers, for instance – attempt to remove obstacles to the achievement of human potential. These obstacles can be biological, educational, environmental, psychological, political, social, institutional, and so on. A surgeon will remove a tumour, a health visitor will attempt to improve housing conditions for a family, and an educator will attempt to remove the obstacle of ignorance and will work to develop powers of reasoning and reflection.

Even traditional health work must often look further than biological understandings of disease. Given that such a wide range of factors can cause disease, even if conventional health work was to concentrate solely on helping people achieve a better physical condition for themselves and others, its subject matter could justifiably include biology, and also such subjects as law, political education, social policy, economics and philosophy. For instance, a health educator who presented only current theories of cancer mechanisms to people who suffered at Bhopal or Chernobyl, or to people living near Seascale in the UK whose houses are excessively irradiated, would be offering a very incomplete service.

But where should the health educator stop? What are the limits to work for health?

This is a perplexing question. In a sense there are no limits to work for health, especially if it is accepted that individuals are each a minute part of the total environment, part of a single vastly complicated whole. However, this will not do for either professional or lay health work. In order to do anything properly we must decide what limits to put on the extent of our tasks.

The **foundations theory of health** can help in this respect. We have discovered that the essence of theories and approaches designed to increase health is to overcome obstacles which face individuals. Work for health must focus on helping individuals, but at the same time be aware that work at the collective level can often be the only way to assist us with our foundations.

Work for health is to do with facilitating individuals to achieve chosen and biological goals, but work for health cannot be limitless – not all work should be thought to be health work. Such a state of affairs is not possible, nor is it desirable to have professional interference in the name of health covering all aspects of individuals' lives. Once suitable background conditions have been created, the achievement of particular chosen potentials should be up to the individual and not the concern of health workers, although permanent maintenance work will often need to be carried out on the foundations.

Work for health is analogous to work needed to lay the foundations of a building. Obstacles such as poor drainage, subsidence, awkward outcrops of rock (analogue: disease, illness, poor housing, discrimination, unemployment) have to be eliminated or overcome in some other way. Then firm foundations and reinforcements have to be added (analogue: good general education, confidence in thinking things through personally rather than relying on what one has been told, good opportunities for self-development). But, unlike the case of building construction, work for health should stop here. What a person makes of his foundations is up to that person, so long as he possesses at least the bones of the *central conditions*. Given this, an individual must be allowed to become the architect of her own destiny.

THE LIMITS TO HEALTH WORK

For practical purposes there have to be some limits to work for health (just as we need a limit to 'roundness' in order to think and act meaningfully using the concept). Health workers must be able to decide on priorities, and to focus on specific targets of primary concern. *The basic limit to work for health is that it must be work on the foundations or set of conditions necessary for the achievement of some biological and chosen potentials. Health work must be intended to enable people to develop themselves – to enable them to work towards the achievement of other biological and chosen potentials.* These potentials should include both body building and intellect building, because people have mental life as well as physical existence.

The set of basic conditions must be of primary concern for health workers, although they must always be aware that, in particular cases, obstacles can be created by unexpected factors. *The key is that work for health is work on building a solid stage, and keeping that stage in good condition. The roles people perform, and how they choose to perform them upon the stage, should be up to the individuals provided that the platform is sound.* For instance, health workers should not interfere once autonomy has been achieved by an individual. It is not the job of work for health to help in the achievement of a great many potentials people may choose, or to prevent the achievement of chosen potentials even if their achievement will undermine the foundations of the individual concerned. In such cases choice is paramount.

The *central conditions* given above are the primary targets in work for health.

The limits to the legitimate meanings of health are intimately connected to the limits to health work. The analogue between 'roundness' and 'health' is not perfect. There is more fuzziness to the limits to health work than to the limits to the meaning and use of the word 'roundness', for the following reason.

Although the central foundations can be stated clearly enough, the needs of particular individuals in particular circumstances can be so diverse that work on laying exceptional foundations may be necessary. For instance, it is not normally the job of a health worker to provide books on specialist subjects, although health workers should ensure that people understand where they can obtain them for themselves. However, if the person they are trying to help is a prisoner and the prison cannot supply these books, then it would be appropriate for a health worker, as part of her professional activity, to furnish the books in order to enable the prisoner to begin personal work to develop himself, since their continued absence may constitute a very significant *liability.*

When the occasion demands, elements which normally lie outside the limit of work for health may enter it briefly. For instance, spending the final hours with a dying person in order to enable that person to achieve better the little potential that is left to him is not part of the normal scope of work for health. The normal area of concern is to do with building and maintaining the basic foundations for individual self-development; however, a substantial part of a health worker's normal role is *vigilance.* She must observe and take note of the times when tasks that are normally not work for health become work for health temporarily.

WHAT ARE THE ANALOGUES OF SOCRATES' SQUARES?

What aspects of life are not normally or not ever the concerns and targets of work for health?

1. *Specific training in specialist subjects*. Work for health does not normally involve training people about building and construction, or engineering, or in foreign languages, or non-basic maths, for example.

2. *Unproblematic everyday normal activities*. For instance, shopping, socialising, and relaxing should not normally concern health workers. A person who is living as a fulfilled member of a society should be left alone by health workers.

3. *Personal choosing when a person has the central conditions* is never to do with health workers.

4. *Health workers should never resort to indoctrination*. Such tactics might be appealing since they can be effective, but indoctrination should be avoided because the long-term effect of its continued use is to undermine some of the central conditions for health.

5. *Health workers should never restrict the information available* to individuals, even when it is contradictory and conflicts. People should be allowed to arrive at their own conclusions.

6. *Health workers should attempt to limit personal choices and potentials only when their fulfilment will undermine the basic foundations of other people*.

7. *Work for health should never cultivate activities that will undermine the foundations of the target individual or group, or which will undermine the foundations of other people*. For instance, work for health should not encourage disease-creating activities, activities which create negative stress, or monotonous, unfulfilling activity. According to the **foundations theory**, work for health can never advocate dismantling foundations for achievement; however, there is an important distinction to be made. In cases where people do things which undermine other people's foundations, it may be appropriate to intervene directly. For instance, if a factory is seriously polluting a neighbourhood, thus undermining many people's biological foundations, then it may be both possible and apt to instigate legal action against the factory owner. However, if an individual who is well aware of the implications of what he is doing to himself chooses to adopt a way of life which undermines some or all of his foundations for achievement, then health workers have less power. They may continue to present information about the consequences of this activity, and may even suggest alternatives, but they can do no more than this, and should stop even this work if requested.

According to the theory that health is equivalent to the state of the set of foundations necessary for personal achievement, the task of all health workers must be to provide as strong a set of foundations as possible, but only some are central and needed by all. Great care must be taken to ensure that other foundations laid are *appropriate* to the chosen potentials a particular person is trying to achieve.

Health workers should constantly reflect on what they are doing when they attempt to promote health. They ought to ask whether a particular person actually wants what the health worker is trying to give him. Perhaps the 'client' smokes 30 cigarettes per day, drinks 5 pints of lager each evening, and habitually eats rich fried food. Yet even the health promoter must ask whether the 'client's' priority is to stop smoking, to moderate his drinking, and to diet – or is he happy doing these things? Will things be worse for him if he does modify his habits? Are there more pressing obstacles in the way of him achieving chosen potentials? Does he want to move to another area? Does he want a garden? Does he not want a garden? Does he want a different house? Does he need a challenge? Does he need some form of intellectual stimulation? What does he prefer? What is the point of lengthy counselling on the dangers of smoking when the person wants to change his life in some other way, enjoys smoking and is prepared to accept the risks?

If this point is accepted, health workers will subscribe to the view that a person should be permitted to choose to undermine some of his or her foundations for achievement. Health workers must accept this conclusion so long as the person understands clearly what he is doing, though this does not mean they must stop spreading ideas in which they believe (so long as they do not present them as morally binding truths, which would be to indoctrinate). Nor does it mean that they must necessarily cease action at a collective level aimed at curbing cigarette and alcohol advertising, production, and consumption, for example (see **Figure 7**).

Although the fullest individual health is achieved when a person is unimpeded in the pursuit both of her chosen potentials and of her biological potentials, choice must be paramount (with the proviso that this choice must be based on personal reflection and consideration of the consequences). People are more than biological units.

ASSESSING THE STATE OF PEOPLE'S HEALTH

According to the **foundations theory of health** it is impossible to evaluate health precisely.

However, it is possible, and very useful for both practitioners and clients, to have some idea how to distinguish different levels of health.

The state of a person's health is dependent on the amount and range of obstacles eliminated or overcome, and on the quality and quantity of the background conditions provided or available. Health is thus equivalent to the amount of freedom of choice and action a person has. If this is true then the level of a person's health is directly related to the strength of her foundations, and at least a loose idea of that person's health is constantly available.

It is not the purpose of this book to develop a full system by which health can be quantified, though it is possible to imagine such a system. For instance, different obstacles to achievement could be given negative values dependent on how serious a liability each is, and different enabling conditions could be given positive values dependent upon how enhancing each is. For example, diseases could be measured dependent upon how disabling they are, how long they persist, and how life-threatening they are. Other liabilities which might be roughly quantified are poor housing, lack of knowledge, and illiteracy, for instance. Such negative weightings could be counter-balanced by the positive values of the features in people's foundations.

This sort of system would be unwieldy and contentious. Certainly, no standards could be proposed without persisting dispute, yet if people are willing to accept a fairly high

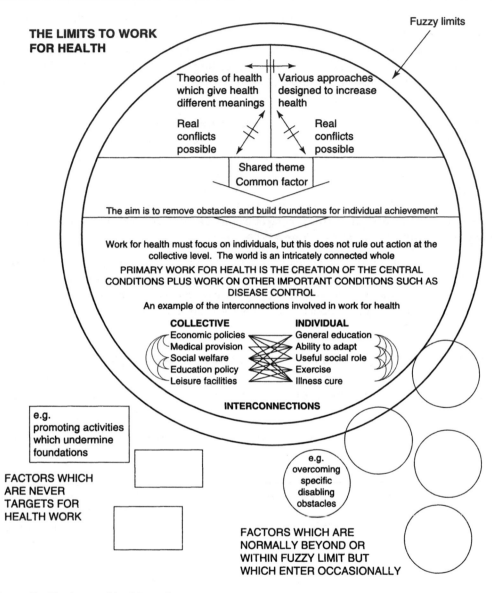

Figure 7   The limits of health work

level of imprecision such a system could provide a practical guide to people's state of health, along a crude continuum as shown in **Figure 8**.

This proposal is different from that intended to measure a person's quality of life in cases where resources for medical treatment are in short supply.[74] That system assumes that positive potentials are as fixed as negative personal circumstances, which is an inexcusable pessimism the **foundations theory of health** is designed to combat. Work for health is work to enable. Consequently, a permanent central question is 'How can we provide more enabling conditions for this individual?'

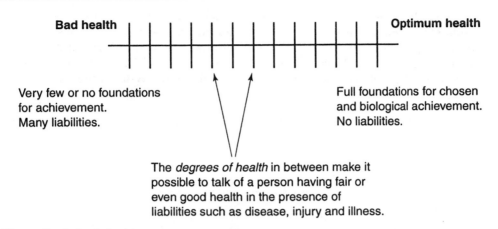

Very few or no foundations
for achievement.
Many liabilities.

Full foundations for chosen
and biological achievement.
No liabilities.

The *degrees of health* in between make it
possible to talk of a person having fair or
even good health in the presence of
liabilities such as disease, injury and illness.

Figure 8   A simple health assessment measure

WHAT IS WRONG WITH THE FOUNDATIONS THEORY?

There are many possible objections to this theory, certainly more than are listed below. Most can be answered, at least in part.

1. *The theory is just one person's idea of health. We have been told that health cannot be defined, and that there can be no universally acceptable theories of health. So this theory is just as good, and just as bad, as any of the others.*

Response

There are no finally objective standards against which to measure the worth of theories, but there are other standards. The **foundations theory** shows where other theories of health are insufficiently thought through; it argues that certain areas should be primary targets for health workers, and it provides a crude way of assessing health – thus it is a gauge for practical work. Furthermore, it is more specific than other theories, and as a result it is easier to show where it slips up, and to suggest improvements. In all these things the **foundations theory of health** is an advance on other theories.

2. *The theory is an argument for political and social change which uses health as a convenient and emotive platform. It is just one more instance of bandwagon jumping.*

Response

The theory is indeed an argument for social change, and can apply to any society.

Health is the focus because so many people work in the name of health, and so much is written about health, without those who do the work and the writing being fully clear about what they are doing or what they mean. The theory does not use health as an emotive platform (though health is inevitably an emotive issue), rather the theory developed from a genuine philosophical compulsion to clarify the meaning of health.

Moreover, people of very different political allegiances can find much to agree with in the **foundations theory**. All political systems attempt to create foundations of some kind for their people. The natures of these foundations, and the method of their creation, tend to be the subject of political dispute. It would be good to have an equivalent level of debate about health priorities, and the **foundations theory** can help bring this about.

3.   *The thinking behind the theory is idealistic. The theory tries to point the way to a utopia.*

Response

In a way this is true, but people should have visions. We need ideals, so long as we realise that this is what they are.

For everyone to have the fullest degree of health possible as unique individuals there would have to be tremendous social, political and economic upheaval. However, most practical work for health does not strive directly for such huge goals. Since work for health focuses on the individual, and recognises that individuals can never be divorced from their wider environments, it is possible to increase health by small degrees. The hope is that these small steps multiply and progress accelerates.

It has been argued by Marxist thinkers and others that there is a contradiction here. It is said that by trying only to help people in small ways health workers 'patch up' the existing social system – they reinforce it by helping people operate again in the very system which created their ill-health in the first place. This objection would be telling if health workers did not at the same time try either to improve existing systems or to change them altogether – which of course they often do. In any case, which is better: to leave people to suffer when you have the power to improve their lives in some way, in the hope that all this suffering will somehow bring about change? or to help people cope within the existing situation, at the same time promoting the idea that the existing system should and could be altered?

4.   *The theory is not fully worked out.*

Response

This is true. The **foundations theory** is developed further in **Chapter Seven** (and has now been expanded in several other texts).[14,51,75] Theories take time to grow. They need to be put to work and criticised.

THE FULLEST SENSE OF HEALTH – UPDATE

This is the book's central chapter, since it introduces the **foundations theory of health**, made more explicit in later works (and see **Figure 9**).

However, its philosophical basis is given in the original chapter (which I have altered as little as clarity will allow). Indeed, it is better to read the theory rather than visualise

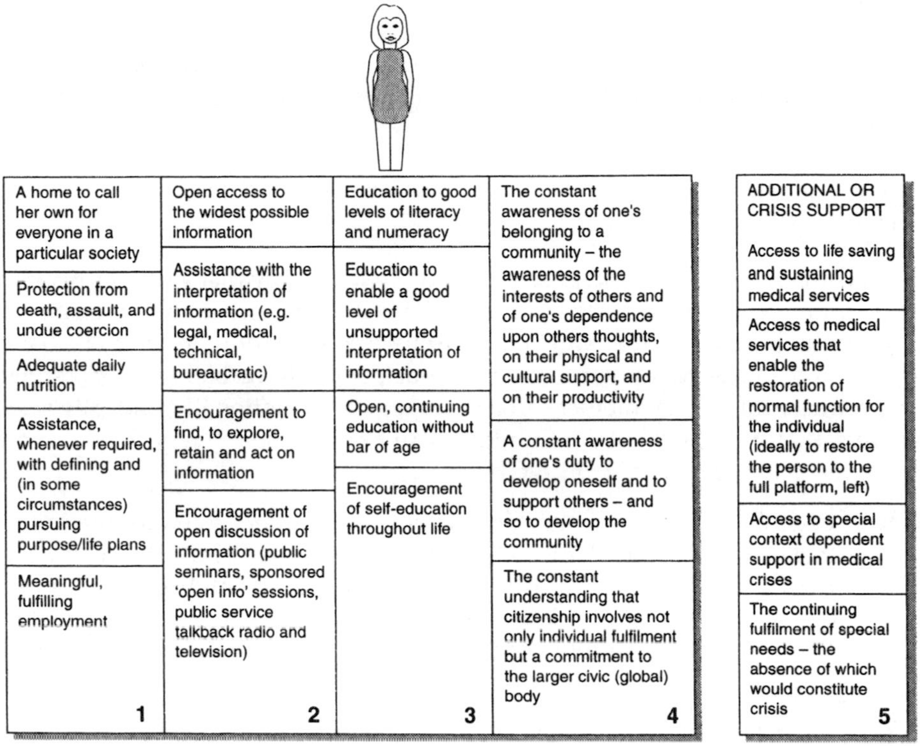

A home to call her own for everyone in a particular society	Open access to the widest possible information	Education to good levels of literacy and numeracy	The constant awareness of one's belonging to a community – the awareness of the interests of others and of one's dependence upon others thoughts, on their physical and cultural support, and on their productivity	ADDITIONAL OR CRISIS SUPPORT
Protection from death, assault, and undue coercion	Assistance with the interpretation of information (e.g. legal, medical, technical, bureaucratic)	Education to enable a good level of unsupported interpretation of information		Access to life saving and sustaining medical services
Adequate daily nutrition				Access to medical services that enable the restoration of normal function for the individual (ideally to restore the person to the full platform, left)
Assistance, whenever required, with defining and (in some circumstances) pursuing purpose/life plans	Encouragement to find, to explore, retain and act on information	Open, continuing education without bar of age	A constant awareness of one's duty to develop oneself and to support others – and so to develop the community	
	Encouragement of open discussion of information (public seminars, sponsored 'open info' sessions, public service talkback radio and television)	Encouragement of self-education throughout life		Access to special context dependent support in medical crises
Meaningful, fulfilling employment			The constant understanding that citizenship involves not only individual fulfilment but a commitment to the larger civic (global) body	The continuing fulfilment of special needs – the absence of which would constitute crisis
1	**2**	**3**	**4**	**5**

Figure 9   The foundations for achievement

it as a stage, because simplified illustrative images (like **Figure 9**) tend to detract from its depth.

AN AMBIGUITY

It may be interesting to note that the foundations' definition of health says:

> A person's (optimum) state of health is **equivalent** to the state of the set of conditions which fulfil or enable a person to work to fulfil his or her realistic chosen and biological potentials.

This was and is what was intended – and is the understanding depicted in **conception three** (see **Figure 3**). A person's health does not **depend** on the foundations, it is **equivalent** to them. However, the original chapter contains two confusions (retained for the most part in this revised version) about the status of the foundations figure.

Ambiguity One – Individuals or Groups?

The original **Chapter Five** states that work for health is work with, for or on individuals. It hardly considers groups at all, and indeed the definition of health begins:

> A **person's** (optimum) state of health is .... (bold added)

If you read an early print of the first edition you will see, just above this definition, that the phrase which appears in the later printings of the first edition (and in this second edition):

> It is a question of providing the appropriate foundations to enable the achievement of personal and group potentials

does not contain the words 'and group'. I thought at the time that work for health must begin and end with individuals because – if I remember correctly – I assumed that only individuals could be the targets of health work, since only individuals have *both* biological and intellectual potential. Groups of people have biological potential (we can reproduce, infect one another, affect one another emotionally and physically by what we say and do), but only individuals can *conceive*, and I very much wanted to promote the *power of conceiving* in the book.

However, even though it is true that groups of people cannot think as one individual can, nevertheless it is obvious (at least it seems so now) that work for health can and should be directed toward groups as well as individuals – both because it is possible and desirable sometimes to enable biological potentials on their own, and because promoting a sense of community (one of the four central conditions for health) is usually best done with groups of people.

I am now clear that the foundations figure can represent one person, two people, a family, a larger group, a nation or everyone in the world. It all depends what the health worker wants and is able to do.

Ambiguity Two – Is the Foundations Figure to be Included in the Assessment of Health Status or Not?

Figure 6 above expresses the original position well. The phrase at its centre sums it up:

> The state of the various background conditions which can enable the achievement of personal potential. The state of a person's health is equivalent to the state of these conditions.

The idea was that health is to do with individuals and that the state of the foundations (boxes 1–5 in **Figures 3** and **9**) simply is the state of a person's health. Assess the amount of information available to a person, assess the state of her basic needs, assess her abilities to assimilate this information, and assess the additional support available, then you assess her state of health.

Taken at its word, this understanding yields a very strange image, a perversion of **conception three**, shown in **Figure 10**.

In other words, on a strict reading of the first edition it looks as if one might assess a person's health without assessing the person physically and mentally – a rather extreme reaction to the expropriation of health by medicine! I did not intend this, but equally I did not pay sufficient attention to the merits of the conventional view (my

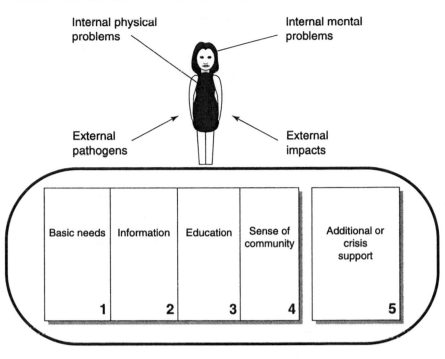

THE STATE OF HEALTH OF AN INDIVIDUAL OR A GROUP

Figure 10   A misunderstanding of the foundations conception of health

philosophical prejudices and enthusiasm for unconventional alternatives held too much sway). The result was an ambiguity that is now plain, but was obscure at the time. For example, within **Figure 6** I say:

> The state of the various background conditions which can enable the achievement of personal potential. The state of a person's health is equivalent to the state of these conditions.

(Note that I also use arrows misleadingly in **Figure 6**, thinking partly in accordance with **conception two**, when of course there should be no arrows, just as there should be no arrows emanating from the foundations platform – see **Figure 3**.)

And on the same page I also give as an example of work for health:

> A surgeon will remove a tumour ...

But I cannot really have it both ways. I believe I imagined I had included a person's physical and mental condition within the first *central condition* (or box 1), but this seems to have been wishful thinking.

I am now clear that any assessment of the foundations figure's health – be it an individual or a group – should include an assessment of the obstacles and potentials present *within* the foundations figure, and therefore that Figure 3 is the correct way to think of the **foundations theory of health**.

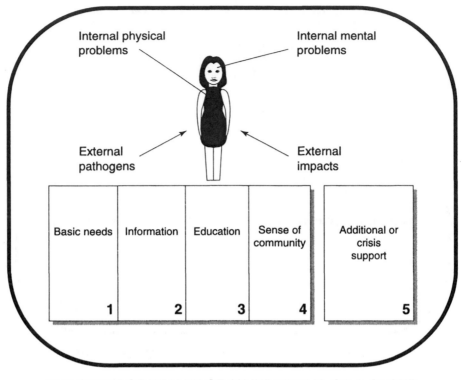

THE STATE OF HEALTH OF AN INDIVIDUAL OR A GROUP

Figure 3   The foundations conception of health

THE SENSE OF COMMUNITY

The fourth central condition has also developed over the years:

> 4. *The recognition that an individual is never totally isolated from other people and the external world.*
> People are complex wholes who cannot be fully understood separated from the influence of their environment, which is itself a whole of which they are a part. People are not like marbles packed in boxes, where they are a community only because of their forced proximity. People are part of their whole surroundings, like cells in a single body (I thank Dr Michael Wilson for these metaphors). This fact compels the recognition that a person should not strive to fulfil personal potentials which will undermine the basic foundations for achievement of other people. In short, an essential condition for health in human beings who are aware of the implications of their actions is that they have an awareness of a basic duty they have because they are people in a community.

In the first edition I believed that this condition rested on the fact that all individuals are connected to other individuals biologically, socially and emotionally, and deduced (rather weakly) a duty on each of us therefore to treat all other people equally. The inclusion of this central condition has always and obviously seemed prejudiced – more so than the other conditions, though they are in fact equally prejudiced (see

Health Promotion: Philosophy, Prejudice and Practice[14]). I have now come to see this condition as less to do with duty *per se* and more to do with an awareness that ought ideally to prompt feelings of duty. For example, in *Health Promotion*, this 'health condition' becomes:

> The constant awareness of one's belonging to a community – the awareness of the interests of others and of one's dependence upon others' thoughts, on their physical and cultural support, and on their productivity.

In other words, if one doesn't have this awareness then one is suffering a major health deficit – an obstacle to health, an obstacle to a fulfilling human potential.

THE PRACTICAL APPLICATION OF THE **FOUNDATIONS THEORY OF HEALTH**

The first edition assumes that the **foundations theory** has applications, the intervening years have demonstrated it. The **foundations theory** can be used:

1. As a way of setting personal health targets
I have developed an online version of the foundations template which can be completed by anyone. A person can fill in the five boxes to assess her present state of health, and can compare these with her depiction of her preferred or even ideal state.[76]

2. As a way of engaging the recipients of health care in the assessment of their state of health and in planning what to do to improve it

For example, consider the following exercise from an online course in health care analysis:

Charles' Stroke – Exercise Two

CHARLES' STROKE

Charles is 80 and has had a right-hemisphere haemorrhagic infarct. He has completely lost the use of his left leg. His right arm and leg are still sound but his left arm and side are very weak. He can speak, but only with great difficulty. It is not easy to understand him. Charles is a retired boiler-maker, well known for being a cheerful, harmless soul. He has two adult sons who both live a couple of car-hours away.

Before his stroke he was living routinely in a council house, with his wife, two years his junior. She (Mary) has always been in charge of the major household decisions. Charles would have liked to have had more of a say, but Mary is a born leader and smarter than him, so Charles gave this ambition up a long time ago. Charles' passion was gardening – he grew prize tomatoes and chrysanthemums – a hobby which kept him happily occupied for much of the day.

Two weeks ago Mary woke to find Charles immobile by her side in their bed, tears running from his eyes. She guessed what had happened straightaway, called the doctor and an hour later Charles was in an ambulance on the way to hospital.

Kate is one of Charles' nurses, and a devoted nurse advocate. At first she wasn't sure whether he would survive, but she can see he is recovering slowly – at least physically. Kate's just heard that Charles' physiotherapy is to be increased, with a view to significant rehabilitation – even to getting him walking again. As she chirpily tells Charles this latest news he fixes her with a brutal glare – 'SSfuck sssthat' he dribbles. Kate is shocked, but Charles forces on. 'I'm sno ussse na. No phhss…no mrre phsssthhry. Fththuuc off.' Then he shuts his eyes.

◆

Kate is an experienced nurse. She thinks it possible that in time Charles may recover enough to be able to walk around the house (and his garden) using a frame. Perhaps he might do even better than this, if he has a will to. Her assessment of Charles' present state of health, using the foundations template, is shown below

Charles

Comfort ——— Reassurance	Information about strokes and their effects	Help to understand the information and make it relevant	Knowledge of other people with strokes and their ways of coping	+	Physiotherapy
1. Basic needs	2. Information	3. Education	4. Sense of community	+	5. Additional support

Figure II   Charles' foundations through Kate's eyes

She assumes that the best way to care for Charles is to be completely honest about everything, including her growing fondness for Charles and Mary and her frustration that Charles will not do what she *knows* to be best for him.

Consequently, Kate shows the foundations image to Charles and explains it to him. She asks Charles if she might also show it to Mary. Charles agrees and they both work out a foundations image.

It turns out that Charles' foundations image (shown below) is radically different from Kate's:

Charles

LEAVE ME ALONE			+	**No more physio.**
1. Basic needs			+	5. Additional support

Figure 12   Charles' foundations through Charles' eyes

And Mary's (shown below) is different again:

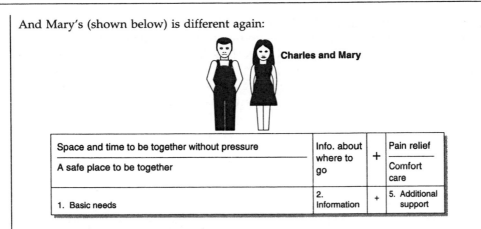

Charles and Mary

Space and time to be together without pressure	Info. about where to go	+	Pain relief
A safe place to be together			Comfort care
1. Basic needs	2. Information	+	5. Additional support

Figure 13   Charles and Mary's foundations through Mary's eyes

Kate emphasised Boxes 2, 3, 4 and 5. Charles selected Box 1 alone – he does not need anything else. However much he gets better he will not be able to be the person he was before. He cannot pursue Charles' life goals any more, so his life has lost its meaning. He would prefer to be left alone with his memories and when nature takes its course he will accept that.

Unlike Charles, Mary sees the target of care (the foundations figure(s)) as the pair of them, a married couple. Because of this it is not for her to express an individual view – however much she would like to cry out that Charles must do what Kate says – but to express a shared view. She wants Charles back as he was but she knows she cannot ever have him back like this. She also knows that the impact on her, Charles and their relationship will be immense if he does have the physiotherapy and eventually comes home to be looked after by her. She says – courageously and with enormous sadness – that she agrees with Charles. It is better for them if Charles does not have the physiotherapy – that way they can be together in this short trouble and then Charles will be gone.

Your Task

Imagine you are Kate, and remain inclined to encourage Charles to undergo the physiotherapy. However, after discussion between the three of you, you agree to work for health from Mary's perspective. This still gives you considerable practical scope, even though it would not have been your ideal choice.

Using the Foundations tool take Mary's basic foundations image and develop it into a strategy.

The exercise offers one simple example of how all concerned in a health care situation might be involved in thinking therapeutically about health status and health goals.

3.   As a way of open and participatory planning of health systems
Using the template, it is possible to involve as many members of the public as a government wishes in the setting of health priorities – it can even be done and assessed online. Members of the public might be asked to complete the template and to adjust the various sections of it to preferred relative proportions. The collective results could be used to decide on resource allocation.

4. As a questionnaire to establish health beliefs

Of course, to ask people to complete the foundations template in a research project to establish their views of health would be to bias their answers in accordance with a particular theory of health. However, since exactly the same comment might be cast against any other questionnaire with the same end in view – including those currently administered by the health establishment – this is hardly a reason not to proceed.

CHAPTER SIX

The Idea of Human Potential

The idea of human potential also requires clarification. 'Potential' is yet one more 'keyword' which, if care is not taken, can generate a verbal smokescreen.

The **foundations theory of health** argues that *a person's health is equivalent to the state of the set of conditions which fulfil or enable her to work to fulfil her realistic chosen and biological potentials*. Roughly this means that if a person has a broad and sound set of conditions which fulfil or enable her to achieve helpful potentials, then her health is good. If the set of fulfilling or enabling conditions is small and the conditions weak, then her health is poor.

Inevitably this explanation raises further questions, in particular *what is meant by 'realistic'?* and *what is meant by 'potential'?*

1. What is Meant by the Term 'Realistic' in this Theory?

The use of realistic may seem like a 'get-out clause', but it is not meant in this way. It might, for instance, be taken to signify that a 'working-class' child from a 'broken home' should accept that the limit on the positive and fulfilling goals he can achieve is low – that he has been given his lot and should be realistic about it.

If this were the proposed meaning then the theory would be sadly pessimistic. Instead, the word 'realistic' is included in the foundations definition of health to make it clear that the **foundations theory** does not aspire to **WHO**'s apparent goal of complete physical, mental and social well-being – the use of 'realistic' is meant to warn against mythical thinking and the pursuit of impossible goals. Moreover, 'realism' refers mainly to biological potential. In order to improve physically a person must be realistic about her present condition, and about the speed and direction of possible change.

To sum up: reference is made to realism in order to make the point that for a person to achieve any potentials a start has to be made from his present state; however, the inclusion of realism is not meant to advocate a fatalistic attitude to life. Although part of any individual's condition rests on many elements intrinsic to that individual, external circumstances – particularly the social environment – can be changed.

2. What is Meant by 'Potential'?

Assumptions are made in any theory, and it best to be as clear as possible about them.

Assumptions

1.   We are not merely living out a pre-determined destiny which we are powerless to alter. Except in extreme instances of illness or external control (such as continuous solitary confinement without external stimulus), people possess an indefinite number of potentials depending upon what we do, and what happens to us. We all have physical and intellectual potential until we die. Although what has already become actual may increasingly affect that which is still potential – what has happened to our bodies will limit us in a physical sense, and what has happened to our minds will limit us intellectually – the potential to achieve a range of possibilities always remains.

This is true even of terminal patients in hospital, even until the time they finally lapse into unconsciousness. Not only do such people have choices about which potentials to achieve for themselves, they also have the potential to influence other people such as their friends, families, and carers. A dying person might be depressed and self-pitying. She might be pathetic. Or she might inspire, set the example she would wish to have set for her, give love and be loved. She might talk to people in a way she has never done before, and she might see them, and they see her, in a different light.

Throughout a human life a person has a host of latent potentials, which in general will decrease with time. Of course they are not all achievable. Much depends upon circumstances. Some doors open, stay ajar for a while, and then close permanently. Sportsmen choose to specialise, so shutting many other sporting doors as they go through one. Sometimes surprising doors open. For instance, many life prisoners take university degrees, thus fulfilling a potential they probably would never have realised had they stayed out of prison.

2.   The **foundations theory of health** takes an optimistic view of life. It assumes people can change themselves and their environments for the better. It assumes they will want to, and that they will wish the improved conditions they enjoy to be enjoyed by others. It assumes that people do not, and certainly do not have to, think of their potentials only in a selfish way.

Can People's Potentials be Assessed?

Folk dictums like 'give me the boy at seven and I'll show you the man', and 'I always knew he'd turn out to be a bad "un" ' have a point. Psychological and genetic research demonstrates that people do have certain attributes and characteristics which remain with us throughout life.[77]

There are, of course, many tests available to assess potential. For instance, doctors can judge the adult height of a child fairly accurately. We have genetic potentials which determine our biological development. IQ tests can be done to determine the ability of parts of people's intellects. Yet nevertheless the potential of a person is not the same as the potential of an engine – where the maximum possible efficiency can be stated. There is, thankfully, a high degree of uncertainty about which potentials people will achieve. Children confidently predicted to be potential 'bad "uns" ' can turn out to be caring people, clergymen, philosophers, policemen, expert fraudsters, or whatever the opposite of 'being a bad "un"'' is thought to be. The child of 7 may have many fixed characteristics, but a study of the 7-year-old will not show what will happen to the man, nor reveal how he will deal with external events in his 'characteristic way'.

Problem: Not All Potentials Are Good

People are potentially evil, senile, diseased, dead, and stupid. We have the potential to be jealous, malicious, and selfish. We can and do injure, abuse, and impede other people. The problem is that if work for health is work to remove various obstacles to the achievement of human potentials, then why should health workers not remove obstacles which prevent the achievement of the kinds of potentials normally regarded as bad?

How Can Positive and Negative Potentials Be Distinguished?

No absolute distinction can be made since questions of value are always disputed. It is, however, possible to put forward a working distinction.

Work for health is concerned with enabling fulfilling achievements and so aims for the achievement of normal or positive potentials. Medicine is intended to help people achieve fulfilling norms. 'Normal bodies' and 'normal children' will develop in certain predictable ways. If they are developing abnormally then steps may be taken to attempt to bring them nearer to a normal state – unless their abnormalities are regarded as desirable in some way.

Interpretations of 'positive potential' will inevitably vary; however, individuals will usually seek to achieve states they believe will enhance their lives in one way or another. For instance, people might aim to improve physically – by exercising, by dieting, by cosmetic surgery, by other surgery – or intellectually – by reading and taking courses of education – or socially, or emotionally. Not all people will see these goals as positive, but we can all recognise personally enhancing potentials and typically set about fulfilling them.

The idea of 'positive potential' can be contrasted with the idea of *liability*. Liabilities (or negative potentials) are problems that act against the achievement of normal or positive potential. For instance, disease and ignorance are both liabilities which can prevent positive potential.

Essentially:

> *Work for health is concerned with encouraging normal and positive potentials because these potentials have the effect of opening up possibilities for achieving more potentials, whereas negative potentials reduce the number of possible potentials.*

Examples of positive potential are higher standards of reasoning ability, greater assimilation of knowledge, and an increased level of ability to develop oneself autonomously. Examples of negative potential are the potential to commit suicide, the potential to be diseased, and the potential to despair.

The Role of Health Workers in the Achievement of Potentials

Obviously health workers should not promote negative, debilitating potentials. Rather they should seek to enable, to widen and increase possibilities for human achievement. Health workers naturally will not wish those they have enabled then to undermine their own foundations, or to undermine the foundations for achievement of others. However, health workers must remember that choice is a central condition, and that their work stops at work on the foundations. Health workers should not look over the shoulder of a person doing a physics examination, attending a job interview, signing a contract for a house, or sealing a business deal. Individual liberty must be respected. Health workers have no right or duty – other than the legal duties of all citizens in some cases – to prevent a person autonomously choosing a potential with which the health worker disagrees, or which the health worker knows will undermine the given or self-created foundations of that person. For instance, if a person is fully aware of the implications of what he proposes to do, and he wishes to abuse his body in some way, then he must be allowed to do so, although work to show him information which might make him change his mind can continue. Work for health is work to provide the basic foundations for achievement, and then to try to maintain these so that a person always has the widest possible choice about which potentials she can achieve.

THE IDEA OF HUMAN POTENTIAL – UPDATE

Though the statement that:

> Work for health is concerned with encouraging normal and positive potentials because these potentials have the effect of opening up possibilities for achieving more potentials, whereas negative potentials reduce the number of possible potentials

may seem circular, it is nonetheless both informative and practically useful. Just like decisions about what counts as health, judgements about positive and negative potentials necessarily involve human values. However, by incorporating the **species-typical theory of health** (according to which medicine endeavours to restore and ensure biological norms) with the **foundations theory**, it becomes possible to identify *positive potentials* as:

a.   species-typical potentials desired by the foundations figure
b.   chosen potentials that increase the number of fulfilling potentials open to the foundations figure, or at least do not reduce them.

It follows that *negative potentials* are normally:

a.   species-atypical potentials not desired by the foundations figure
b.   chosen potentials that decrease the number of fulfilling potentials open to a person.

These potentials cannot all be specifically detailed in advance. However, the general idea should be sufficient guide to health workers in most cases.

ETHICS IN FOUNDATIONS

Perhaps surprisingly, there are very few explicit references to ethics in *Foundations*, even though, as a colleague noted:

> I thought the whole thing was about ethics.

Accordingly, readers may be interested to note the specifically ethical declaration contained in the chapter's last paragraph:

> Health workers have no right or duty – other than the legal duties of all citizens in some cases – to prevent a person autonomously choosing a potential with which the health worker disagrees, or which the health worker knows will undermine the given or self-created foundations of that person.

This is a clear moral assertion, in the Western liberal tradition: people who know what they are doing should be left alone unless they are harming others. This is famously known as the 'harm principle', usually attributed to J. S. Mill, who wrote the following in *On Liberty*:

> ... the sole end for which mankind are warranted, individually or collectively, in interfering with the liberty of action of any of their number, is self-protection. That the only purpose for which power can be rightfully exercised over any member of a civilised community, against his will, is to prevent harm to others. His own good, either physical or moral, is not sufficient warrant. He cannot rightfully be compelled to do or forbear because it will be better for him to do so, because it will make him happier, because, in the opinion of others, to do so would be wise, or even right... The only part of the conduct of anyone, for which he is amenable to society, is that which concerns others. In the part which merely concerns himself, his independence is, of right, absolute. Over himself, over his own body and mind, the individual is sovereign.[78]

Importantly, in *Health: The Foundations for Achievement* this principle is not simply co-opted from Mill, nor is it merely a taken-for-granted social assumption, rather it stems from the **foundations theory of health** itself. Since the whole point of work for health is to provide *enabling conditions* – foundations that avoid or help people to avoid obstacles to fulfilling potentials – then work for health becomes a *self-limiting* endeavour. The better the health worker does her job the quicker the person achieves health and – as a direct consequence – the less right the health worker has to coerce a recipient to make a decision or to prevent her making what the health worker considers to be a bad decision. Both as a matter of morality (or prejudice, if you prefer) and as a matter of logic – work for health is work to provide potentials which allow people to create and act on as many further fulfilling potentials as possible.

CHAPTER SEVEN

The Assessment of the Health of Individuals

Two questions are considered in this chapter. *Which of the case studies is healthy and which unhealthy?* and *How could each case study become more healthy?*

WHICH OF THE CASE STUDIES IS HEALTHY?

This question was left unanswered at the end of **Chapter One**. The result of the initial inquiry was – and was meant to be – perplexing. Not one of the hypothetical people discussed was unanimously judged to be healthy, and Dennis, Anne, Mr James and Peter were each described as healthy twice and unhealthy twice. The medic, the social scientist, the idealist, and the humanist could not agree, because they hold different ideas about the nature of health.

It is a mistake to think a person's state of health can be precisely measured. There are far too many contestable variables involved, but if work for health is to mean anything it must be possible to have some idea how to appraise it. Furthermore, it is not the case that either a person is healthy or not. People and circumstances are infinitely variable, and so health must be assessed in degrees.

As we have seen in **Figure 8**, health can be thought of as a continuum which takes account of a host of factors.

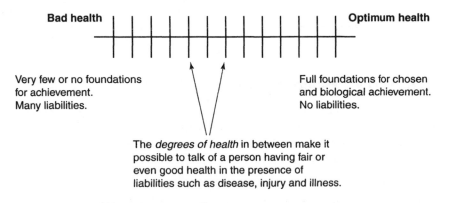

Bad health ⟶ **Optimum health**

Very few or no foundations for achievement. Many liabilities.

Full foundations for chosen and biological achievement. No liabilities.

The *degrees of health* in between make it possible to talk of a person having fair or even good health in the presence of liabilities such as disease, injury and illness.

Figure 8   A simple health assessment measure

The foundations are not all fixed requirements. The general idea can be applied to anyone, even though we have different needs.

This vagueness must be accepted. Not to do so is worse than not being able to measure health at all. Nevertheless, it is possible, by using the **foundations theory**, to state a person's level of health in broad terms. It is also possible to state to what extent one person can have better health, either in general or in a particular respect, than another.

AN ASSESSMENT OF THE STATES OF HEALTH OF THE CASE STUDIES

Assessment can be made to establish which foundations enable to what degree, to see what obstacles are present, and to discover what liabilities need to be removed.

CASE ONE

PERCY

Percy is the ex-office worker who, for the last three years, has been suffering from occasional temporary involuntary delusions during which he believes and acts as if he is another person. When he suffers these delusions he cannot interact normally with other people, and as a result finds it very hard to hold down a job.

Percy has a low level of health. He has not been lucky. His persistent delusions are a major *liability*. They present a large obstacle in the path of a number of potentials he might have chosen to fulfil. However, he does have some health. He has several solid foundations for achievement. He has warmth and shelter, he has a lot of information available to him, he understands his problem and is trying to do something about it. If he found anyone else with a similar problem he would do what he could to help him too. The trouble is that Percy is unable to build on the foundations he has, because of this one huge obstacle.

How Can Percy's Health Be Improved?

Obviously, the impediment must be eliminated. Some way must be found to rid Percy of his curse. If it is found, or if the problem disappears spontaneously, then Percy will need help with another central condition, which we all require anyway. He will need to be helped to recognise a purpose in his life.

If this could be done then Percy's level of health would increase dramatically.

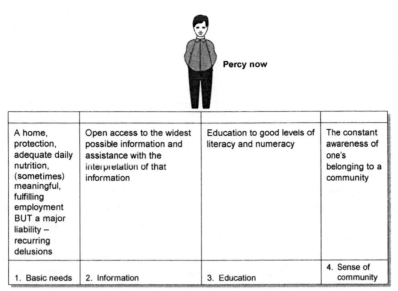

Percy now

A home, protection, adequate daily nutrition, (sometimes) meaningful, fulfilling employment BUT a major liability – recurring delusions	Open access to the widest possible information and assistance with the interpretation of that information	Education to good levels of literacy and numeracy	The constant awareness of one's belonging to a community
			4. Sense of community
1. Basic needs	2. Information	3. Education	

This image shows that Percy has good access to information and is well educated. He also has some needs met. Part of Box 1 represents damage caused by his delusions. Note too that he has no additional or crisis support at the moment.

Figure 14   Percy now

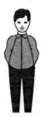

Percy after health work

A home, protection, adequate daily nutrition, meaningful, fulfilling employment BUT a major liability – recurring delusions	Open access to the widest possible information and assistance with the interpretation of that information	Education to good levels of literacy and numeracy	The constant awareness of one's belonging to a community	+	ADDITIONAL OR CRISIS SUPPORT
			4. Sense of community	+	5. Additional support
1. Basic needs	2. Information	3. Education			

In this image Percy still has the liability, however he has been assisted to find a job – as a gardener – where its impact is likely to be minimised. His new employer is fully aware of his condition.

Percy has also joined a mental health support group (and so his sense of community has expanded), and is receiving additional support from his new GP and a community mental health nurse, who has been assigned to him.

Figure 15   Percy after health work

CASE TWO

DENNIS

Dennis is the lazy, apathetic bank clerk. He is not diseased and does not feel ill. He spends his time at the work he has been doing for the last 20 years, watching television, or sleeping.

Dennis' case shows that decisions about a person's state of health can often be hotly disputed (and this has been my consistent experience over the 15 years I have used Dennis as a case study when teaching about the philosophy of health). If Dennis truly wants to live the way he does then he has all the foundations necessary for the fulfilment of his chosen potential. His biological potential does not seem to be seriously threatened by his life-style. It could be argued that Dennis has a high level of health. Alternatively, it could be said that his level of health is fairly low. The problem with Dennis may be that he does not realise what other potentials he has, that he needs stimulus and wider information about what else he could be doing in order to ensure that he has a greater purpose in life.

How Can Dennis' Health be Improved?

If he does not possess this wider information then he might be shown a range of possibilities he could choose to do instead of continuing to idly drift. There are countless fulfilling ways in which he could spend his spare time. However, if he does possess extensive information about choices open to him, and yet still prefers to live as he does, then there is nothing further that can or should be done for him at present.

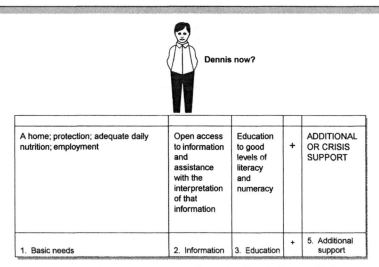

Dennis now?

A home; protection; adequate daily nutrition; employment	Open access to information and assistance with the interpretation of that information	Education to good levels of literacy and numeracy	+	ADDITIONAL OR CRISIS SUPPORT
1. Basic needs	2. Information	3. Education	+	5. Additional support

It is not easy to agree on Dennis' present state of health, but this in itself is a useful discovery.

Here is one possible depiction of Dennis. As can be seen from the relative sizes of the boxes, it assumes that his home life is central, that he has limited information and education, and that he receives occasional support from State health services.

There are many alternative depictions. If possible a health worker interested in enabling Dennis should try to have him complete the template – and ideally ask Dennis' wife to do so too.

Figure 16   Dennis now?

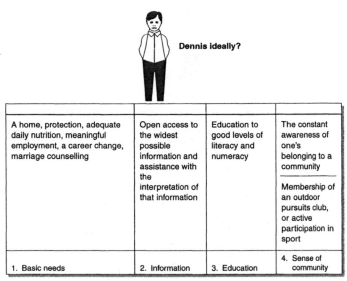

1. Basic needs	2. Information	3. Education	4. Sense of community
A home, protection, adequate daily nutrition, meaningful employment, a career change, marriage counselling	Open access to the widest possible information and assistance with the interpretation of that information	Education to good levels of literacy and numeracy	The constant awareness of one's belonging to a community Membership of an outdoor pursuits club, or active participation in sport

Some health promoters might see this as a more healthy Dennis, others might disagree.

Figure 17   Dennis ideally

CASE THREE

ANNE

Anne is the journalist suffering from paraplegia. Her body was shattered in a car accident, yet she has managed to rebuild her career. She has a warm and convenient flat. She has become reconciled to her disability, is now content, and always tries to encourage other people with their lives and projects.

Anne has a very high level of health even though she is severely handicapped. She has all the *central enabling conditions*, as well as other important foundations, such as her specially designed flat and her assured income, that enable her to achieve her chosen and biological potentials.

How Can Anne's Health Be Improved?

Anne has a full and appropriate set of enabling conditions at the moment. She has sound foundations for achievement which are enabling her to fulfil her realistic chosen and biological potentials.

The notion of realism is very important here. If her handicap could be cured, which is not likely, then Anne would regain a very important and enabling foundation, but she knows her injury is permanent. It is now part of her and she must accept it. If she continued to hope unrealistically, if she fantasised about a return to the way she was, then this wishful thinking would itself become a liability. Her regrets and false hopes would be an obstacle to the achievement of the many positive potentials she still has.

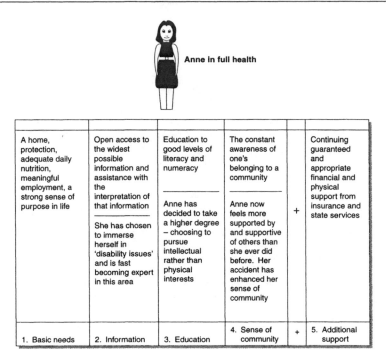

Anne in full health

1. Basic needs	2. Information	3. Education	4. Sense of community	+	5. Additional support
A home, protection, adequate daily nutrition, meaningful employment, a strong sense of purpose in life	Open access to the widest possible information and assistance with the interpretation of that information She has chosen to immerse herself in 'disability issues' and is fast becoming expert in this area	Education to good levels of literacy and numeracy Anne has decided to take a higher degree – choosing to pursue intellectual rather than physical interests	The constant awareness of one's belonging to a community Anne now feels more supported by and supportive of others than she ever did before. Her accident has enhanced her sense of community	+	Continuing guaranteed and appropriate financial and physical support from insurance and state services

Figure 18   Anne in full health

CASE FOUR

BETTY

Betty is the widow with secondary cancer of the brain. She is miserable, frightened, and very worried about the behaviour of her youngest son, but she has great character and is fighting her disease with all the strength she has.

Although Betty has a serious disease she is not totally unhealthy. She has several degrees of health. She has warmth, shelter, and a purpose in life. She understands what is happening to her body and is well educated in other respects. She also cares deeply about what happens to her son. She has a number of foundations on which to build, and one major liability – her cancer.

How Can Betty's Health Be Improved?

Clearly Betty's level of health would improve if her cancer were to be cured, or if she had a remission of the disease. In this case the medical profession has a legitimate and important interest in an individual's state of health. But nothing is ever totally good or totally bad. Even cancer has some benefit. It has brought out a side to Betty – her character and strength – which neither she nor her son realised she had.

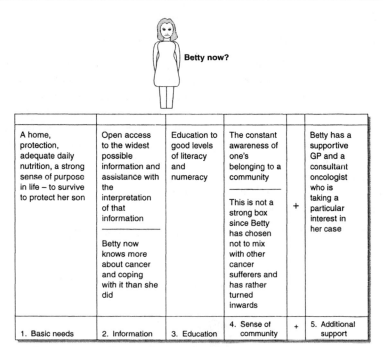

1. Basic needs	2. Information	3. Education	4. Sense of community	+	5. Additional support
A home, protection, adequate daily nutrition, a strong sense of purpose in life – to survive to protect her son	Open access to the widest possible information and assistance with the interpretation of that information ⎯⎯⎯ Betty now knows more about cancer and coping with it than she did	Education to good levels of literacy and numeracy	The constant awareness of one's belonging to a community ⎯⎯⎯ This is not a strong box since Betty has chosen not to mix with other cancer sufferers and has rather turned inwards	+	Betty has a supportive GP and a consultant oncologist who is taking a particular interest in her case

Betty has a reasonable level of health, but her movement on her stage is restricted by her internal liability – her cancer. Could her health be further improved?

Figure 19   Betty now?

CASE FIVE

THE JAMES FAMILY

Mr and Mrs James are the couple, both 20 years old, living in damp conditions, currently without electricity. Mrs James is pregnant and in despair. She has no disease. Mr James does not have a disease either, but is on probation and cannot get a job. Their child has a low level of speech ability for his age, and suffers bronchitis and temper tantrums.

Collectively the family has a poor level of health, and each member considered individually has a poor level of health. Many important foundations for achievement are missing. The family has shelter but no warmth, and little purpose in life. They have very limited access to the information about the factors shaping their lives, and they do not know how to assimilate this information, or how to use it for their benefit. They feel isolated and, understandably, are concerned only to improve their own lives, if possible.

continues

continued

How Can the Health of the James Family Be Improved?

Radical action is called for. The family has numerous latent positive potentials and could be enabled to achieve them. They need electricity and a warm, dry place to live. They need to be shown how to cope better with their money, their relationships, and with contraception. Above this they need a good general education, in addition to information about such things as bronchitis and the dangers of Valium. They need to know many things they currently do not, including the reasons why their flat was built in the first place, and why Mr James cannot find work. They need to understand more about what is happening to them in order to be able to try to do something about their lives. The child needs special attention with his speech, and Mr and Mrs James need to be shown how to enable the child to fulfil more of his potentials.

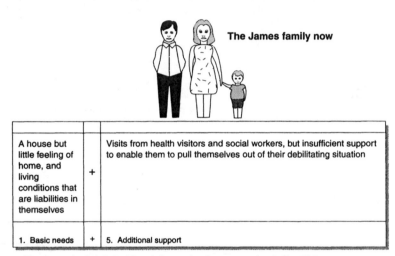

The James family now

A house but little feeling of home, and living conditions that are liabilities in themselves	+	Visits from health visitors and social workers, but insufficient support to enable them to pull themselves out of their debilitating situation
1. Basic needs	+	5. Additional support

The James family's limited foundations – they have a poor level of health but many untapped internal potentials. They need stronger foundations to release these potentials.

Figure 20   The James family now

CASE SIX

WINSTON

Winston is the young, unemployed Maori who lives right next to a busy motorway intersection. He is part of a local gang and is peripherally involved in Maori activism – protesting against colonisation and lack of opportunity for Maori youth. He boosts his income by dealing in 'soft drugs'. He is in excellent physical condition.

continues

─ *continued* ─

As with Dennis, the state of Winston's health is highly debatable. It could be argued that he is fulfilling a high level of physical potential, and that he has most of the central conditions at least in part, and so should be considered to have a fairly high level of health. On the other hand it could be said that Winston has much potential which he cannot currently fulfil because of the prejudice he suffers because of his ethnic background.

How Can Winston's Health Be Improved?

Many of his potentials cannot be tapped because of the obstacles posed by the prejudice of some police and some employers against Maori people.

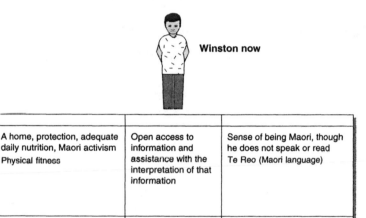

Winston now

A home, protection, adequate daily nutrition, Maori activism Physical fitness	Open access to information and assistance with the interpretation of that information	Sense of being Maori, though he does not speak or read Te Reo (Maori language)
1. Basic needs	2. Information	4. Sense of community

Is Winston as healthy as possible? He is well placed physically to use the limited stage he has – would a bigger and more varied stage enable him further?

Figure 21   Winston now

CASE SEVEN

PETER

Peter is the successful businessman who enjoys a very high standard of living according to Western yardsticks. He smokes and drinks quite heavily, and is often frustrated and loses his temper.

continues

---

continued

Peter is well educated and well housed, and he does care about the welfare of some other people. He has all the *central conditions* to a degree, and he also has other important foundations for achievement. He chooses to smoke and drink, knowing the possible unfavourable implications of his habits. He is not diseased.

Consequently he has a high level of health. He has firm foundations on which to build his next chosen potentials, although he may be undermining the foundations of his biological potential through his lifestyle and his stress.

This is not to say that the more money a person has the more health he has necessarily, however it is a fact that in a capitalist society people need a certain amount of money in order to fulfil much of their potential. Not enough information has been given about his relationship with his wife for his violence to have a bearing on this assessment.

How Can Peter's Health Be Improved?

Once again opinions will vary and be arguable. Value judgements cannot be avoided in health issues.

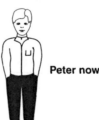

Peter now

A home, protection, adequate daily nutrition, meaningful, fulfilling employment	Open access to the widest possible information and assistance with the interpretation of that information	Education to good levels of literacy and numeracy	The constant awareness of one's belonging to a community
1. Basic needs	2. Information	3. Education	4. Sense of community

Peter has a good level of health. He is bolstered – made confident and assertive – by his affluent lifestyle. He does not have a particularly strong sense of community, though he enjoys his golfing and political friends.

Figure 22   Peter now

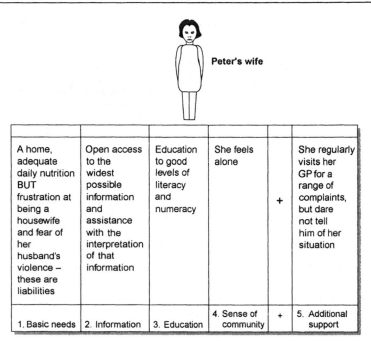

A home, adequate daily nutrition BUT frustration at being a housewife and fear of her husband's violence – these are liabilities	Open access to the widest possible information and assistance with the interpretation of that information	Education to good levels of literacy and numeracy	She feels alone	+	She regularly visits her GP for a range of complaints, but dare not tell him of her situation
1. Basic needs	2. Information	3. Education	4. Sense of community	+	5. Additional support

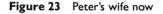

Her stage is much narrower than her husband's – so her health is less [

Figure 23   Peter's wife now

CONCLUSION

Any assessment of people's health according to the **foundations theory of health** will be controversial, even though in many respects the theory is not new at all. It is now well known that a person's way of life can influence his chances of becoming diseased and ill, and it is surely only one or two plausible steps further to say that *a person's health is intimately linked with his quality of life.*

The method of assessment based on the **foundations theory** has advantages over alternatives:

1.   It makes concrete a way of thinking positively about health, and goes further than the idea that health is the absence or the opposite of disease.

2.   It focuses attention on wider aspects of people's lives, rather than concentrating only on conditions and cures recognised by medicine. There is an emphasis on ways of improving health more comprehensive than those proposed by established health services. The **foundations theory** also highlights ways to prevent disease and illness.

3.   It enables health workers to identify the most significant life targets to be changed. Health workers can readily assess which are the most serious obstacles to remove, and which are the most essential enabling conditions to provide (usually and ideally in partnership with the people they are trying to help).

4.   It further illuminates the vast and unnecessary inequalities of opportunity (and so of health) which continue to blight human society.

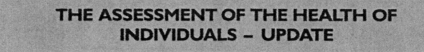

THE ASSESSMENT OF THE HEALTH OF INDIVIDUALS – UPDATE

It may be interesting to note that:

1.   Assessing health in this way shows just how much the foundations idea differs from the health is the opposite of disease theory of health.

2.   The foundations image is limited in the following ways:

   a. While positive foundations can be shown it is not possible to display liabilities, other than by restricting or removing relevant boxes. It is impossible to display a 'negative stage' because almost everyone – whatever their condition or situation – will have some degree of health.
   b. It is difficult to depict the presence and extent of the internal conditions of the foundations figure (the figure's biological and mental state), and sometimes these conditions will be central factors in the figure's health. However, the internal conditions can be readily explained in words. Moreover, better and more flexible foundations images are possible and in development.

CHAPTER EIGHT

The Aims of Health Education and Promotion

INTRODUCTION

The funding of health education and promotion programmes continues to increase,[79] and it is now possible to study for all manner of certificates and degrees in the field. Subjects offered typically include communication skills, social policy, environmental health, social medicine, public health, epidemiology, psychology, sociology, organisation studies, statistics and research design. As far as promoting health in its fullest sense is concerned, such courses – and the work of many qualified health educators and promoters – are inadequate. Despite the good intentions of the health promotion industry, the strategies fall short on two counts:

1.   Although the various theories discussed in **Chapter Four** are widely known, and it is generally acknowledged that health is a very wide 'concept', the practical effect of health education is still to concentrate almost exclusively on preventing diseases, illness and injury. Health educators try to inform people about smoking, alcohol, and drug abuse; about 'foot health' and 'dental health'; about safety in the home and at work; and about the benefits and dangers of physical exercise. These topics are important – and there is no reason why these and similar ideas should not be explained and promoted – but they are only a limited part of true health education.

2.   The theme of current health education and promotion is *prevention*. Yet since a person's health is inextricably linked to her quality of life, the first aim should be to *create*.

Creation is in any case the best form of prevention since creating foundations for achievement can, for example, prevent ignorance, abusive social systems, and the waste of innumerable personal potentials and talents. People are complex, unique, profound, and always important, however unfortunate their current circumstances. But we are not always permitted the right foundations on which to build ourselves. Without these foundations people can be shaky, incomplete, and liable to collapse.

Present health education and promotion works to prevent at a less than fundamental level, rather like trying to dam a stream halfway down a mountain instead of at its source. Logically, the main aims of health education and promotion must be to provide most of the central conditions presented in **Chapter Five**, particularly conditions 2, 3, and 4.

WHAT IS EDUCATION?

Although the nature of health has been clarified in this book, no attempt has yet been made to elucidate the character of education. This will not be attempted in any detail here because, unlike the case of health, there have been philosophical debates about the nature and goals of education since the times of the ancient Greeks.

The question is as difficult and complex as 'What is health?' Nonetheless it is possible to make a simple distinction between the notions of *training* and *education*.

TRAINING

Training is a process that involves imparting related sets of ideas. Training is proper and necessary in disciplines such as computing, engineering and medicine, where correct techniques and formulae must be learnt. Indeed, the importance of a thorough training in practical disciplines cannot be overestimated, however *only* to train where human values, lives, and goals are concerned can be profoundly damaging.

EDUCATION

True education is a process which aims to achieve two principal goals:

1.   To provide the learner, either directly or indirectly, with all relevant information about a subject area.

2.   To retain or re-instil a childlike curiosity; to encourage a questioning attitude, a confidence to select and to criticise; to promote the sense that the information presented is what we have now – but is not the final word; and to encourage the idea that each of us is part of a continuing inquiry. True education enables a person by cultivating his skill to choose autonomously. Simply to present information, theories and techniques is mechanics. It is not education but a form of programming.

If both these goals are aimed for then – given the inevitable real-world limits to autonomy, such as legal rules and the interests of other human beings – it is possible to educate people to be autonomous. It is possible to educate people to the point where they realise that their opinions, theories and experiences are important not only to themselves but also to other people. It is, in other words, possible to educate people to the point where they regain their natural philosophical ability.

Naturally there are many problems with this point of view, however, this is not the place to discuss them.

HEALTH EDUCATION SHOULD NOT INDOCTRINATE. IT SHOULD NOT BE A PROPAGANDA EXERCISE

1. *Indoctrination undermines the central requirements (Boxes 2 and 3) that people should have the fullest possible information about factors which affect their lives, and should have sufficient ability and skills to make their own reasoned choices.*

A useful means of illustrating this point arrived in the mail a few years ago (a drop in the ever-expanding ocean of health promotion propaganda). It was a 'Heart Chart' sent out by members of a 'Well-Man Centre'. The Centre wanted to help people live 'healthier lives', meaning that it sought to help them increase their physical fitness and maintain biological norms.

The chart was intended to help people avoid heart disease. It displayed a 'traffic-light' warning system. A green light meant all was well, an amber light was a warning to change some 'life-style factors', and the red light meant 'stop some habits altogether'. Ten factors which can contribute to or help prevent heart disease (according to the chart) were listed, including smoking, drinking alcohol, eating fried foods, and exercising. Dependent on a person's habits – perhaps she exercises once a week, has little or no stress, and so on – points could be allocated. The best score for each of the 10 categories was 0 and the worst 4. If the total score was less than 10 then a person got a green light, between 10 and 20 he received an amber light, and between 20 and 40 the stop sign 'lit up'.

The thinking behind the chart was presumably well meaning, but the chart gave little useful information, and so was of limited help (at best) in supporting personal choice. Why should smoking increase heart disease? What are the statistics? I'm half the size of my brother so should I eat less fried food than him? We've never had any heart trouble in our family so should I heed these warnings? These are reasonable questions which ought to be answered in any serious attempt to educate.

The 'Heart Chart' is an archetypal example of the dangers of not giving sufficient information, and therefore of attempting propaganda. Without further information the reader may be seriously misled. In fact, the chart's 'programming' was so awry the reader could smoke 80 cigarettes a day and get thoroughly drunk every night, score 0 on the other 8 factors, achieve a total score of eight and so get a green 'traffic light'.

Childhood immunisation campaigns are also and undoubtedly meant to indoctrinate. A comparison of the leading (state sponsored) websites in favour of immunisation and those against (community initiated) speaks for itself.[80,81] The better anti-immunisation sites not only cast significant doubt on the establishment's claims, they provide access to scientific papers and *adverse immunisation events reporting systems* rarely if ever mentioned in official literature aimed at encouraging patients to vaccinate their children. Even if it is true that on balance it is better that children are immunised, it is not better for the public's foundational health that such a distorted representation of reality is patronisingly put forward as the incontrovertible truth.

2. *Opinions about even the traditional subjects of health education are divided. There is always a degree of uncertainty, and people should be made aware of this.*

Professor Michael Oliver, the then President of the British Cardiac Society, reinforced this point in August 1985. He rejected the idea that low fat diets can save people from heart attacks. In Oliver's view public health campaigns to reduce the death toll caused by heart disease by changing lifestyles nationwide are simplistic. Professor Oliver agrees that smoking is a factor in heart disease, but argues that once smoking is excluded most people who suffer coronary disease have none of the other supposed risk factors in significant proportion to those who do not have coronary disease. The causes of heart disease seem to be diverse, and their analysis and understanding is complicated and uncertain. All the causes of heart disease may not be known, and those which affect one person's heart need not affect another person's heart. He was quoted as saying:

> Such is the force of the juggernaut that has been set forth by these propagandists that little credence is given to genuine scientific doubts. Much of the zeal has arisen from the enthusiasts allowing themselves to be coerced.
>
> Many health professionals ignore, and some are ignorant, of alternative approaches to coronary heart disease. We must go on with some forms of health education campaigns, but there are many other things to consider.[82]

Professor Oliver has a clinical specialist's interest in, and view of, health, but he makes a sound general point. Educating, promoting, or working in other ways for the health of others, and working for an individual's own health, is never a matter of following fixed policies or given rules without thinking. Smoking, eating butter, or drinking alcohol regularly, are not activities which are unequivocally anti-health. For instance, Bill Werbeniuk, who was a fairly well-known snooker player in the 1980s, claimed to need 14 pints of lager beer a day in order to play to the best of his ability (ironically to stop his hands shaking), a potential to which he gave higher priority than the physical well-being of his liver. It is also true that smoking can ease nervousness and tension, and can help with camaraderie.

People must be allowed to exercise choice, and the fullest choice can come only from possession of the fullest relevant information.

THE CENTRAL AIMS OF FOUNDATIONAL HEALTH EDUCATION

These should be:

1. *To ensure that all people have a good standard of general education.*

The philosopher Paul Feyerabend wrote:

> ...one thing must be avoided at all costs: the special standards which define special subjects and special professions must not be allowed to permeate general education and they must not be made the defining property of a 'well-educated man'. General education should prepare a citizen to choose between the standards, or to find his way in a society that contains groups committed to various standards, but it must under no condition bend his mind so that it conforms to the standards of one particular group. The standards will be considered, they will be discussed, children will be encouraged to get proficiency in the more important subjects, but only as one gets proficiency in a

game, that is, without serious commitment and without robbing the mind of its ability to play other games as well. Having been prepared in this way a young person may decide to devote the rest of his life to a particular profession and he may start taking it seriously forthwith. This 'commitment' should be the result of a conscious decision, on the basis of a fairly complete knowledge of alternatives, and not a foregone conclusion.[83]

Feyerabend exhorts us to provide *central conditions* for health as a prerequisite for citizenship. This is the real challenge for health education. If such a state could be achieved universally then we would be blessed with a shifting, vivacious, exciting, free society.

To disregard Feyerabend's pleas is to be accessory to the sacrifice of a latent genius possessed by all of us, and to sacrifice the creative spirit present even in the 'living statues' described by Oliver Sacks on the altar of conservatism, tradition, mediocrity, and fixed order. Not to provide these essentials is to deny choice, and as such is the asphyxiation of morality. The key to health is to allow people to develop themselves.

2.   *To develop people's powers of conceiving, and so to enable them to make the most of the information they have.*

JOHN BERGER'S OBSERVATION OF THE DEPTH WHICH ALL PEOPLE HAVE

The writer John Berger is concerned about the poverty of the human condition. In his book, *A Fortunate Man*,[84] he relates some of the experiences of John Sassall, a fictional country doctor – created by Berger from observation of real life cases – who meets birth, suffering, and death as part of his daily work. Sassall feels empathy with his patients but, although he is glad to have his own fortunate circumstances, he feels frustrated that only he amongst the community in which he practises possesses the words and education necessary to articulate his thoughts and so protest about the emptiness and powerlessness of the human lives he encounters. It is not that people do not have the potential to be able to live fulfilled lives, rather they have not been given the linguistic tools they need in order to make sense of their experiences and their conceivings. Not the least of Berger's points is that the way society (in his case British society) is constructed acts to waste and empty most of the lives it does not destroy.

Berger acknowledges that in order to realise a more full and equal achievement of human potential it is vital that all people should practise and become proficient in conceiving in the widest possible way, and so learn to select from a range of theories in response to unique situations and experiences, rather than act according to set dictates:

> Good general diagnosticians are rare, not because most doctors lack medical knowledge, but because most are incapable of taking in all the possible relevant facts – emotional, historical, environmental as well as physical. They are searching for specific conditions instead of the truth about a man which may then suggest various conditions. It may be that computers will soon diagnose better than doctors. But the facts fed to computers

will still have to be the result of intimate, individual recognition of the patient. (pp. 73–74)

One of Berger's points is that computers are limited by the theories they are given. Such theories may be very good diagnostic tools, but they are not the whole story about diagnosis. Human involvement and the ability to empathise are required as well. The best healers must pick up clues and hints, respond personally, come to know and understand other human beings by being able to imagine themselves in the position of those others.

Berger is talking about the power of conceiving. A power that needs theories but which also goes beyond theory:

> There are large sections of the English working and middle class who are inarticulate as the result of their wholesale cultural deprivation. They are deprived of the means of translating what they know into thoughts which they can think. They have no examples to follow in which words clarify experience. Their spoken proverbial traditions have long been destroyed: and, although they are literate in the strictly technical sense, they have not had the opportunity of discovering the existence of a written cultural heritage. (pp. 98–99)

These people can conceive but they cannot translate their ideas into words and action. Without a 'cultural literacy' there is usually no route from the conceiving, to the concept, to a theory and so to practice. Without having had access to an education which goes beyond standard literacy and numeracy, without anything more than a superficial knowledge of theory and language 'ordinary people' are deprived of a full opportunity to assess and to debate both inwardly and outwardly. Of course they have life experience, and practical and intuitive skills, but they do not have the means to develop this knowledge into communicable theories of life:

> What I am saying about Sassall and his patients is subject to the danger which accompanies any imaginative effort. At certain times my own subjectivity may distort. At no time can I prove what I am saying. I can only claim that after years of observation of the subject I believe that what I am saying, despite my clumsiness, reveals a significant part of the social reality of the small area in question, and a large part of the psychological reality of Sassall's life. *The greatest stumbling block to accepting this is the false view that what people cannot express is always simple because they are simple. We like to retain such a view because it confirms our own bogus sense of articulate individuality, and because it saves us from thinking about the extraordinarily complex convergence of philosophical traditions, feelings, half-realised ideas, atavistic instincts, imaginative intimations, which lie behind the simplest hope or disappointment of the simplest person.* (p. 110) [Italics added]

This argument is the opposite of elitism. Berger is describing the unique and remarkable human ability of conceiving, the possession of which indicates the great depth of human beings – even of the ones regarded as 'simple' or 'thick', or any other of the many unkind labels we tend to use. There is great scope for development if only people are given the opportunity – the right circumstances for growth. It is not naïve idealism to argue that people should be given the chance to develop themselves to the full – on the contrary, it is the only civilised course to take.

THE LIKELY BENEFITS OF THESE CENTRAL AIMS

The reason why we should educate for and promote health is to lay foundations for self-development in a world of vastly complicated interconnections.

The Benefits for 'Lay-people'

Given the wider knowledge, competence, and confidence necessary for increased self-development there will be:

1.   Less feeling of worthlessness.

2.   An ability and an inclination to educate other people – to assist others to the stage where they can begin, at whatever level, to develop themselves.

3.   The practical opportunities to debate 'health issues'. In other words people will be able to discuss their own and other people's qualities of life in wide terms.

As far as problems of illness and disease are concerned there will be:

1.   Far less need for paternalism by doctors. The reflex response – illness symptoms so, a visit to the doctor so, blind obedience of the doctor's instructions – will be replaced by informed conversation resulting in personal choice.

2.   Less dependence on the traditional health services. Those capable of self-care and self-development will demand to look after themselves, if they possibly can. As a result there will be less crowded surgery waiting rooms, and reduced hospital waiting-lists.

The Benefits for Health Care Professionals

An appreciation of the arguments put forward here will not only benefit 'lay-people'. The whole range of present health care professionals will gain. Although they will retain their specialist skills they will also recognise that they have a wider, more generalist role. The general emphasis of their work will change – the broad focus will be on how to encourage and assist people to develop themselves. And the most significant benefit of all for the health professional will be *intellectual liberation*.[51]

An Illustration of this Point from Health Visiting*

*A health visitor is a qualified nurse with further specialised training, experienced in child health, health promotion and health education. Her job is to help people 'stay healthy and avoid illness'. Health visitors work with all age groups.

Unique situations confront health care professionals constantly. Like all health workers, health visitors frequently have the opportunity to make personal informed judgements, but are often constrained by set rules and procedures. How, for instance, would a health visitor react to the many problems presented by the James family (pp 9–10)?

Is the problem medical, environmental, social, psychological, or something else? Is it all of these things? Where does the health visitor begin to offer solutions? There are no clear rules to follow in such cases as this – different health visitors may well opt for different courses of action. And this is a good thing.

Health visiting draws on a range of disciplines because health visitors aim to remove obstacles to people's potentials in their home and family environments. Health visitors learn theories of nutrition, sociology, social policy, psychology, epidemiology, and child development – and in addition must be qualified nurses – but there is no systematic rationale of health visiting or the teaching of it. Consequently there is a debate in health-visiting circles about the need for a comprehensive theoretical model of health visiting to which all tutors, fieldwork teachers, and practitioners could subscribe. This lack of a coherent model concerns some health visitors who have become accustomed to doing what they have been told. It frightens people who are assured by rules.

John Stuart Mill made telling comments on the topic of rule following:

> Thus the mind itself is bowed to the yoke: even in what people do for pleasure, conformity is the first thing thought of; they like being in crowds; they exercise choice only among things commonly done: peculiarity of taste, eccentricity of conduct, are shunned equally with crimes: until by dint of not following their own nature they have no nature to follow: their human capacities are withered and starved: they become incapable of any strong wishes or native pleasures, and are generally without either opinions or feelings of home growth, or properly their own. Now is this, or is it not, the desirable condition of human nature? (p. 119)[78]

The fear and disorientation experienced by some health visitors is made worse when, as often happens in practice, the various specialist theories are in conflict. Should the James child be given medication and the parents counselled, or should the child be removed from such a poor environment? Should the Jameses be rehoused, or should they be shown how to get things changed on their own behalf? Should Mr James be made to do community work instead of his probation, or should something be done about getting him a proper job? How is the health visitor to choose the most appropriate course of action in such a complex case in the absence of guiding theory? The Council for the Education and Training of Health Visitors puts the problem in this way:

> Much literature relevant to health visiting is descriptive; very little explains how to do health visiting. Principles are implied but rarely examined or made explicit. For this reason theories and methods taught can only be ... (those) ... of individual tutors based on their own personal experience. Lack of security in health visiting theory is a problem for fieldwork teachers who have the explicit responsibility of correlating theory with practice. How can I correlate theory with practice for a student when neither of us seems to know what the theory is?[85]

(See *Practical Nursing Philosophy: The Universal Ethical Code*[75] for the answer)

It is at such points that the power of conceiving – which is often simply called 'commonsense' – is invoked to synthesise such elements as theories, empathies, past experience, discussions with colleagues, and common humanity. What is missing is not competence but individual confidence to shake off a debilitating reverence for specific theories and rules. As things stand health visitors are often confused, uncertain, and lack confidence. They feel they are doing wrong by not following set prescriptions for action and as a result can, because they feel they have to, invoke preferred specific theories which seem the least irrelevant in given situations, but which, because they are specific, may not produce the best results. Many health visitors do not have the confidence to take an overall view of their practice. They look at a situation and are taught to make lists of single aims and objectives, when they really need a wider, more flexible and fluid approach, constantly bearing in mind their fundamental enabling role. The central question for health visitors should always be 'How can I enable this individual or family best, how can I get them to the point where they can work to develop themselves?' Certainly specific obstacles – such as the bronchitis and the damp – will need to be eliminated but these obstacles should not be thought of in isolation from the wider problem. Health is equivalent to the set of conditions which fulfil, or enable an individual to work to fulfil, his biological and chosen potentials. How to create better health is never clear-cut – this basic point should never be forgotten. By splitting the task of health creation into specific domains and objectives there is a real danger that the wider aim will be neglected. Theories must be used, but they should not be used apart from the power of conceiving.

Dingwall has argued:

> Doctors don't worry about a theory of medicine; engineers don't worry about a theory of engineering. They follow courses which the practitioner may then use in a personal synthesis to meet the demands of any individual situation.[86]

The other benefits for present health care professionals, whatever their specialism, are that they will recognise the need to add to the width of their conceiving. Since their careers are dedicated to the removal of obstacles to the achievement of human potential they should work to understand more theories, and to gain more experience relevant to their wide vocations. Unless good reasons are advanced to show this to be counter-productive, this recognition will lead to a breakdown, or at least a blurring of, the demarcations between specialisms.

The final benefit will be that health workers will come to understand that they are essentially educators. In all cases of contact with clients, theories, alternatives, consequences and choices should be explained. This may be time-consuming in the short term, but if practised always and universally will have significant long-term benefits.

SUMMARY AND CONCLUSIONS

The aim of health education and promotion is, in general, to bring the individual – and so to bring groups of individuals – to the level where they have the best sets of background conditions for his, her or their chosen and biological potentials. Health education and promotion is about creating choices (and certainly not just those choices preferred by the health promoters themselves). Health education should go further than is traditional, both in the training of the health educators and in the education they provide to others in turn. Full health education is not just to do with creating traditional health choices about such things as smoking and exercise, and it is not only to do with creating choices at the level of a one-to-one relationship with a client. Education for, and the promotion of, health goes far wider than this.

1.   At the individual level health education is to do with making people as fully aware as possible about the factors which can affect their basic foundations for achievement. Because of this, full health education must ensure that people understand the causes of disease and illness, but also that they are politically literate – that they have a knowledge of the institutions and policies which shape their lives. If people have poor levels of general education then health education should work to remedy this.

Health education should also teach people to face questions directly, and to think for themselves. It should aim to develop people's powers of conceiving. Education for health is work for wholeness. It is not just to do with physical functioning, it is at least equally to do with the mental life of a person. It is misleading to speak of 'health potential' or 'health status' with their present limited meaning. This usage tends to focus attention solely on biological potential, but work for health in its full and proper sense is work towards laying the foundations for full human flourishing. This is what a true health service should be aiming to do. The removal of the obstacles of illness and disease is only one aspect of true work for health. True health education should work to enable people to understand better what they are, what they believe, and what they know. It should seek people's opinions and it should enable discussion. The last thing health education should do is to treat people like babies. People are tremendously complicated and often devastatingly underdeveloped. People need to be challenged. We need to be forced to face our worlds.

As Mill has written:

> The human faculties of perception; judgement, discriminative feeling, mental activity, and even moral preference, are exercised only in making a choice. He who does anything because it is custom makes no choice. He gains no practice either in discerning or in desiring what is best. The mental and moral, like the muscular powers, are improved only by being used. (pp. 116–117)[78]

2.   Just as full health education has to involve political education and not indoctrination, health promotion has to involve political action. 'Health for All' will not have been achieved even in a situation where all members of a society have optimum physical fitness if other foundations for the achievement of potential are weak, and other human potentials restricted.

The acknowledgement that political literacy and action are a part of work for health should not be thought to be the pollution of an otherwise pure discipline. Traditional health care is not removed from politics. For example, political ideals underlie the continuing tensions between public health services and the private provision of medical care. Decisions about the funding of national health services are taken by politicians. Political decisions are taken about the roles of medicine and health education. Not to provide a more positive and comprehensive service is both overtly and tacitly a political act. To maintain the present system in the face of alternatives is a political decision.

There are so many factors which influence people's basic foundations for achievement. Such factors as racial discrimination, unequal distribution of income and power, inadequate housing, a poor education service, and low levels of fulfilling employment all have a significant bearing on the quality of people's lives. Promotion and education for health consequently involves explaining and publicising these influences, highlighting particular problems, suggesting alternatives, pressing for change, writing articles, writing letters to the press, and pushing these ideas amongst other professionals.

This task should not fall only on those of one political belief. There is room for many different ideals in health creation. It may be that people who incline towards the political Right will be less keen and less able to do these things. But, if they are truly to work for health, if they are to create equitable foundations for achievement, then this is what they must do. To argue that eventually the best foundations will be laid by getting rid of all foundations – by doing such things as dismantling the welfare state, by providing only basic vocational training, by cutting state benefits, and by cutting the funding of present enabling services – so that the strongest will flourish, create wealth, and then hand some of it back to those who do not have foundations, is immoral, selfish nonsense. It is immoral because there can be no morality without choice, and to remove all foundations is effectively to remove all meaningful choice from many people. It is selfish because it permits unfettered self-interest at the expense of others. And it is nonsense because the habitually self-motivated cannot, and do not wish to, make a sudden conversion to the sacrifices – in money, in time, and in thinking about other people – involved in caring for and providing the basic needs of others.

THE AIMS OF HEALTH EDUCATION AND PROMOTION – UPDATE

Readers should note that the above discussion has been extensively elaborated and superseded by *Health Promotion: Philosophy, Prejudice and Practice.*[14] However, in keeping with my aim to preserve the innocent zeal of the first edition, the chapter has been retained, mostly in its original form. It is, essentially, an appeal for health promotion and education to concentrate first on the *central conditions* (or foundations) for health rather than on the special problems of disease and illness. Were health promoters to do this then they would seek first to promote general literacy and reasoning abilities – so to enable people to work out how to live for themselves – rather than invent ways of encouraging or coercing people to avoid disease. Thus – in line with the book's general position – the chapter proposes a radical redirection of health promotion – the key question becomes not 'How can I change these people's behaviours?' but 'How can I promote the most unfettered conceiving?' I suggest the latter question is fundamental.

CHAPTER NINE

How Can Health for All be Achieved?

This should not be the final chapter, but the first. The question requires, and has received throughout history, considerable thought and argument. In one sense the answer is simple. How can health for all be achieved? Answer: such a state can never be achieved. Health for all cannot be had because Utopias cannot be attained. Different people have different values and priorities and so we will never agree on what counts as Utopia. Furthermore, people inevitably suffer, are sick, and have countless other problems. The world is such that there will always be winners and losers – consequently health for all is a hopeless dream.

In another sense the answer to the question is vastly complicated, and of course depends on what is meant by 'health'. How can health for all be achieved? Answers: by revolutions – bloody, intellectual, or some other kind. By democratic processes – by slow change from within. By direct political action to redistribute wealth and power. By extending true education. By changing rigid, de-energising social institutions. By legal reform. By economic change. By group pressure. By working to extend people's imagination. By some combination of all or some of these answers. It makes sense to propose these answers so long as health is seen according to the **foundations theory** advanced in this book. If a person's health is equivalent to the state of his set of foundations for achievement, then the issue is not 'How can Utopia be created?' but 'How can *equitable minimum conditions to enable people to achieve fulfilling lives* be created? How can the *central conditions* which make up health be best provided for all people?'

The drive to create health for all is not fundamentally to do with the meanings of words, though conceptual analysis should never be allowed to slip into the background. Rather the practical debate must take place at the level of political and social theory and policy. It cannot be denied that people possess a great range of potentials, the question is *what system will bring the most of them to fruition*? And this question spawns a million others: where will the money come from? Who is to suffer and who is to impose the sacrifices which will inevitably be required of some people? What degree of coercion is permissible in order to bring about ultimately liberating changes? Can defence and medical spending be cut to provide an improved education service? Should single societies aim to create the minimum conditions, and then work to help other societies, or should work for health be constantly global?

There is a seemingly endless minefield of theoretical and policy dilemmas to negotiate. These have to be considered and explained, and decisions have to be reached, but it should never be forgotten that now, in the real world, millions of people are shamefully ignorant, underdeveloped, badly fed, badly housed, and saturated with indoctrination. Analysis and discussion should not conceal the need for action now, at whatever level, aimed to improve the health of all people, whether they are friends, neighbours, strangers, or enemies. There is always something, however small, that can be done to enable someone to achieve more than otherwise would have been the case. This is what matters most. We need to think deep, hard and long, to work out ways of providing more of this liberating service.

CONCLUSION

Although this inquiry has endeavoured to understand more about the meaning of health, and of the implications of different theories of health, it has also tried to lay a foundation of its own. Unless it is seriously mistaken, the **foundations theory of health** demonstrates that work for health is inevitably controversial and never a matter of following ordained guidelines unthinkingly. *Work for health inescapably requires thought and reflection about which course of action is the most appropriate in any situation which seems to require some sort of assistance.* Therefore, work for health in itself should create more health in the workers.

This book has tried to bury the myth that the goal of 'health for all' is solely or primarily the concern of medical science. Medicine should be seen as one way, amongst many others, of working to create health. It is not necessarily the most important.

This is a major logical consequence of the **foundations theory of health**, the argument for which only scratches the surface of an intensely complex (almost certainly not fully penetrable) problem about how to improve the quality of human existence. However, as far as ideas directly about the nature of health are concerned, at least it scratches deeper than has been scratched previously. So many controversies arise out of the book, there are so many unanswered questions, and so much has not been properly thought through, that it is plainly inadequate. But in some places it is stronger than others and it is here that any critics should concentrate. If health is not to do with the quality of human life then what is it to do with? If health is properly and exclusively the concern of medicine and para-medicine, why is this so?

References

1. Bates, E. & Lapsley, H. (1985). *The Health Machine: The Impact of Medical Technology*, Penguin Books, Australia.
2. Rimal, R. N., Ratzan, S. C., Arnston, P. & Freimuth, V. (1997). Reconceptualizing the 'patient': health care promotion as increasing citizens' decision-making competencies. *Health Communication*, **9**(1), Hillsdale, NJ, Lawrence Elbaum.
3. Williams, R. (1976). *Keywords*, Fontana/Croom Helm, London.
4. King, L. S. (1954). What is disease? *Philosophy of Science*, **21**, 193–203.
5. Seedhouse, D. F. (1998). *Ethics: the Heart of Health Care* (2nd edn), Wiley, Chichester.
6. Wittgenstein, L. (1974). *Philosophical Investigations*, Basil Blackwell, Oxford.
7. Monk, R. (1991). *Ludwig Wittgenstein: The Duty of Genius*, Vintage, London.
8. Partridge, E. (1966). *Origins*, Routledge & Kegan Paul, London.
9. http://www.yourdictionary.com/cgi-bin/mw.cgi?dlookup=WHOLE&dib.x=1
10. http://www.yourdictionary.com/cgi-bin/mw.cgi
11. Foucault, M. (1973). *The Birth of the Clinic* (translated from the French by A. M. Sheridan Smith), Tavistock, London.
12. Bacon, Francis. (1620). *Novum Organum*, Book I, Aphorisms 1–68.
13. Bacon, Book XLII, Aphorism 42.
14. Seedhouse, D. F. (1997). *Health Promotion: Philosophy, Prejudice and Practice*, Wiley, Chichester.
15. Bacon, Book XLIV, Aphorism 44.
16. Solzhenitsyn, A. (1971). *Cancer Ward*. English translation © (1969), Bodley Head, London, pp. 467–468.
17. Gallie, W. E. (1964). *Philosophy and the Historical Understanding*, Chatto & Windus, London, p. 189.
18. Polanyi, M. (1973). *Personal Knowledge*, Routledge & Kegan Paul, London, p. 4.
19. Staniland, Hilary. (1972). *Universals*, Doubleday/Anchor, Garden City, New York.
20. Koestler, A. (1969). *The Act of Creation*, Hutchinson, London.
21. Kovacs, J. (1998). The concept of health and disease. *Medicine, Health Care and Philosophy*, **1**, 31–39.
22. Culver, C. M. & Gert, B. (1982). *Philosophy in Medicine*, Oxford University Press, New York, p. 65.
23. Diamandopoulus, G. T. (1996). Cancer: an historical perspective. *Anticancer Research*, **16**, 1595–1602.
24. White, W. A. (1926). *The Meaning of Disease*, Williams & Wilkins, Baltimore, MD.
25. Peery, T. M. & Miller, F. N. (1971). *Pathology* (2nd edn), Little Brown, Boston.
26. Field, D. (1976). The social definition of illness. In D. Tuckett (ed.), *An Introduction to Medical Sociology*, Tavistock, London.
27. Manu, P. (ed.) (1998). *Functional Somatic Syndromes. Etiology, Diagnosis and Treatment*, Cambridge University Press, New York.
28. Elliot, C. (2000). Pursued by happiness and beaten senseless: Prozac and the American Dream, *Hastings Centre Report*, **30**(2), 7–12.
29. http://www.britannica.com/bcom/eb/article/4/0,5716,118054+10,00.html
30. Cohen, D. (1989). *Soviet Psychiatry: Politics and Mental Health in the USSR Today*, Paladin, London, p. 24.

31. http://www.psych.ucsb.edu/research/cep/index.html
32. Dubos, R. (1959). *The Mirage of Health*, Harper & Row, New York.
33. Parsons, T. (1981). Definitions of health and illness in the light of American values and social structure. In A. L. Caplan, H. T. Englehardt, Jr & J. J. McCartney (eds), *Concepts of Health and Disease: Interdisciplinary Perspectives*, Addison-Wesley, Reading, MA, p. 69.
34. Seedhouse, D. F. (1994). Health values or business values? *Health Care Analysis*, **2**(3), 181–186.
35. Sacks, O. (1982). *Awakenings*, Picador, Pan Books, London.
36. http://www.humanism.org.uk/
37. http://qb.soc.surrey.ac.uk/resources/keyvariables/macintyre.htm
38. Herzlich, C. (1973). *Health and Illness*, Academic Press, London.
39. Williams, R. (1983). Concepts of health: an analysis of lay logic. *Sociology*, **17**(2), 185–205.
40. Calnan, M. (1987). *Health and Illness: the Lay Perspective*, Tavistock, London, ch. 2, Lay Conceptions of Health Threats.
41. Blaxter, M. (1990). *Health and Lifestyles*, Tavistock/Routledge, London, ch. 3, What is Health?
42. D'Houtard, A. & Field, M. G. (1986). New research on the image of health. In C. Currer & M. Stacey (eds), *Concepts of Health, Illness and Disease: a Comparative Perspective*, Berg, Oxford, pp. 235–255.
43. Crawford, R. (1984). A cultural account of 'health': control, release and the social body. In J. B. McKinlay (ed.), *Issues in the Political Economy of Health Care*, Tavistock, London, pp. 60–103. (Abridged version in A. Beattie et al. (1993), *Health and Wellbeing: a Reader*, Macmillan, London, pp. 133–143.)
44. Mansfield, K. (1977). *Letters and Journals*, Pelican Books, London.
45. Illich, I. (1977). *Limits to Medicine*, Pelican Books, London.
46. Downie, R. S., Fyfe, C. & Tannahill, A. (1990). *Health Promotion: Models and Values* (1st edn), Oxford University Press, Oxford.
47. Black, D. (1982). *Inequalities in Health: The Black Report*, Penguin, Harmondsworth.
48. Acheson, D. (1998). Independent inquiry into inequalities in health reports, Stationery Office, ISBN 0-11-322173-8.
49. Mitchell, J. (1984). *What Is to be Done about Illness and Health?* Penguin, Harmondsworth.
50. Gorz, A. (1983). *Ecology as Politics*, Pluto Press, London.
51. Seedhouse, D. F. (1991). *Liberating Medicine*, Wiley, Chichester.
52. Aguirre-Molina et al. (1993). Health promotion and disease prevention strategies. *Public Health Reports* (Sept.–Oct.), **108**(5), 559–564.
53. Dr Rosemary Biggs, personal communication.
54. Illich, I. (1971). *Deschooling Society*, Harper & Row, New York.
55. http://www.jcn.com/humanism.html
56. Nelson, D. (1997). *Spirituality and its place in the philosophy of health*. Masters thesis, University of Auckland.
57. Boorse, C. (1977). Health as a theoretical concept. *Philosophy of Science*, **44**, 542.
58. Boorse, C. (1987). Concepts of health. In Van der Veer, D. & Regan, T. (eds), *Health Care Ethics: An Introduction*, Temple University Press, Philadelphia, p. 371.
59. Dom Felice Vaggioli. (2000). *History of New Zealand and its Inhabitants*, Otago University Press.
60. AIDS Research Review (passim). AIDS Research Information Center, Inc., 20 South Ellwood Avenue, Suite 2, Baltimore, MD 21224-2241.
61. Nordenfelt, L. (1993). *Quality of Life, Health and Happiness*, Avebury Press, Aldershot.
62. Tengland, P. A. (1998). *Mental Health: a Philosophical Analysis*, Department of Health and Society, Linkoping University.
63. Durie, M. H. (1985). A Maori perspective of health. *Social Science and Medicine*, **20**, 483–486.
64. Ngata, P. & Dyall, L. (1984). Health: a Maori view. *Health*, **36**, 2.
65. Durie, M. H. (1994). Maori perspectives in health and illness. In J. Spicer, A. Trlin & J. A. Walton (eds), *Social Dimensions of Health and Disease: New Zealand Perspectives*, Dunmore Press, Palmerston North.
66. Barwick, H. (1992). *The Impact of Social and Economic Factors on Health*, Public Health Association of New Zealand, Wellington.

67. Whitbeck, C. (1981). A theory of health. In A. L. Caplan, H. T. Englehardt, Jr & J. J. McCartney (eds), *Concepts of Health and Disease: Interdisciplinary Perspectives*, Addison-Wesley, Reading, MA.
68. Wilson, E. O. (1975). *Sociobiology: the New Synthesis*, Belknap Press, Cambridge, MA.
69. http://www.who.int/hpr/cities/index.html
70. http://www.who.int/mental_health/pages/about.html
71. Breggin, P. R. (1994). *Toxic Psychiatry*, St. Martins Press, New York.
72. Wittgenstein, L. (1968). *Philosophical Investigations*, trans. G. E. M. Amscomb, 3rd edn, Basil Blackwell, Oxford.
73. Seedhouse, D. F. (1985). Nurses' Concepts of Health, Wolverhampton Polytechnic (unpublished survey).
74. McKie, J., Richardson, J., Singer, P. & Kuhse, H. (1998). *The Allocation of Health Care Resources: an Ethical Evaluation of the 'QALY' Approach*, Dartmouth, Aldershot.
75. Seedhouse, D. F. (2000). *Practical Nursing Philosophy: the Universal Ethical Code*, Wiley, Chichester.
76. http://online.aut.ac.nz/learnon/588807/course.nsf (enrolled students only).
77. Brody, N. & Ehrlichman, H. (1997). *Personality Psychology: the Science of Individuality*, Prentice-Hall, Englewood Cliffs, NJ.
78. Mill, J. S. (1910). *Utilitarianism, On Liberty, and Considerations on Representative Government*, Dent, London.
79. Le Fanu, J. (1994). *Preventionitis: the Exaggerated Claims of Health Promotion*, Social Affairs Unit, London.
80. http://www.cdc.gov/nip/vacsafe/
81. http://www.new-atlantean.com/options.htm
82. The Cholesterol Scare has been Overplayed. *The Times*, 10 January 1996.
83. Feyerabend, P. (1978). *Against Method*, Verson, London, pp. 217–218.
84. Berger, J. & Mohr, J. (1976). *A Fortunate Man*, Writers and Readers Publishing Cooperative, London.
85. Council for the Education and Training of Health Visitors (1997).
86. Dingwall, R. (1977). *The Social Organisation of Health Visitor Training*, Croom Helm, London.

Index

Note: page numbers in *italics* refer to figures

Aberdonians, elderly 50–1
achievement 131
adaptability of humans 51–2
adaptation
    ability 53
    autonomous 51
    changing circumstances 81–2
    positive 53
    process 59
AIDS 68
alcoholism 39
allergy 39
ambiguity of words 26
anti-immunisation websites 123
antibiotics 60
anxiety 54
apathy case study 8, 11, 12, 112, *113*
autonomy 3
    achievement of potential 105, 106
    carer 61
    choice of potential 107
    clarification 19
    collective action 60
    decrease with modern medicine 58, 59,
        60
    education 122
    enhancement by medicine 60
    healthy state 74
    personal 59
    subordination to medicine 58

Bacon, Francis 25–7
bad health notion 51
Berger, John 125–6
biological potential 95, 96
    health education/promotion 129
    paraplegic case study 113
    realism 103
Black, Douglas 53
Boorse, Christopher 67, 68

cancer 52, 54
cancer patient 9, 11, 12, 13
    work for health 114, *115*

carer, autonomy 61
catatonia 49
categories of health 74–80
change
    desire for 45
    life targets 119
children
    immunisation campaigns 123
    as philosophers 17–18
    rebellion 20–1
choice
    denying 125
    exercising 124
    informed discussion 127
    morality 131
citizenship 125
clarification 16–17, 19, 20
clarity
    thought 25
    word definitions 28
collective action 60
colonial influence on Maori 70
colonisation, infection exposure 68
commodity theory of health 39, 40, 41, 45,
        47–53
    conceptions of health 79
    medical assumptions 55, 67
commonsense 128
community
    central condition for foundations theory
        98–9
    place of individuals in 85–6
competence, self-development 127
competition 52
conceiving 35
    act of 32
    health education 130
    human factors 33
    meaning 29, 32–4, 36
    personal 33
    power 126, 128, 129
    promotion 131
concept(s) 35
    articulation 31
    cultural literacy 126

concept(s) (*cont.*)
  evolution 32
  external description 31
  external reference 31
  of health 50
  meaning 29, 30–2, 35–6
  mind 32
  personal 31
  personal experience 32
  potency 31–2
  problems 31–2
  theory relationship 35
conceptions of health 74–80
confidence
  health visitors 128–9
  self-development 127
Council for Education and Training of Health
    Visitors 128
creation of health 87, 121, 129, 133
  ideals 131
  medicine 134
creative act 33
creative spirit 125
cultural literacy 126
cultural skills 70, 72
Culver, Charles 37, 38

Daniels, Norman 67, 68
death, patterns of 54
definition, meaning of 29, 30, 35
degrees of health 83
delusions 7–8, 11, 12
  state of health 110, *111*
democracy 28
depression 9–10, 11, 12, 55
  personal relationships 87
  work for health 115–16
Descartes, René 32
desirability of health 6
deviation from norm 38
diagnosis 125–6
dictionary definitions 5–6, 23–5
Dingwall R. 129
disagreement acknowledgement 82
disaster relief workers 6
discomfort feelings 39
disease 37–41
  absence 55
  biological understanding 87–8
  causes 66
  concept 6
  control 39
  definitions 38–9
  diagnosis 38
  discovery of causes 52
  eradication 39
  health notion 51
  liability 105
  measurably abnormality 39
  obstacle removal 130
  pattern 37
  power of overcoming 50–1

prevention 119, 121
  psychological reaction 39
diversity, human 63
doctors
  health definition 11–12
  paternalism 127
dogmatism 17
domestic violence 11, 12
  work for health 117–18, *119*
drug dealing 10, 12, 13
  work for health 116–17
drugs, possession 45
Dubos, René 43, 51–2
Durie, Mason 70, 72
duty to get better 44

economic policies 66
education 122
  goals 122
  health care workers 129
  political 130
  see also health education
emotions 57
enablement 84, 92, 107
  factors for health 74
  paraplegic case study 113
encephalitis lethargica 48
epidemics, modern medicine 58, 59
epidemiological research 56
ethics
  in foundations theory of health 107
  meta-ethics 16
evolution concept 32

family 61
  wellbeing 70, *71*
fear of remaining alone 26, 27
Feyerabend, Paul 124–5
Field, David 39
fitness necessary to perform normal tasks 39,
    40, 41, 44–5
  conceptions of health 79
focus in human thought 25
foot-binding in China 6
Foucault, Michel 24–5
foundational health education, central aims
    124–9
foundations theory of health ix, 36, 68, 69,
    83
  ambiguities 95–7
  assumptions 103
  Caroline Whitbeck's theory 73–4
  central conditions 85–8, 89, 97, 98–9, 133
  correct interpretation 97, *98*
  development 36
  ethics 107
  groups 95–6
  health assessment 119–20
  human potential 103–7
  ideals 94
  internal conditions 120
  liabilities 89, 120
  mental condition 97

objections 93–4
optimism 104
physical condition 97
practical application 99–102
similarities to Maori theory 70, *71*, 72
social change 93–4
species-typical theory of health
    incorporation 106
freedom of choice 91
fulfilling life, achievement 133
funding allocation 78

Gallie W. B. 29, 34
germ theory 52
Gert, Bernard 37, 38
goal seeking 52
golden age, mythical 61
Gorz, Andre 55
groups, foundations for health 95–6

hale, meaning 24
hallucinations 7–8, 11, 12, 49
    state of health 110, *111*
happiness 74
    goal 46
harm principle 107
healers 126
health
    absence of disease 55
    common factor of approaches 63–7
    conceptions 1–4
    contemporary medical understanding 1–2
    desirability 6
    enabling factors 74
    as end 63
    foundations xiii
    foundations concept 3–4
    history of term 23–5
    ideal 81–2
    meanings xi, xii, 5–6, 23–7
    as means 63
    measurement 83
    personal assessment 12
    philosophical investigation 13
    quantification 56, 57
    semantics 13
    social and environmental circumstances
        2–3, 4
    uses of term 5
    WHO definition 41–3
health beliefs questionnaire 102
health care, medical view 36
health care workers 86
    achievement of potentials 106
    benefits of foundations theory aims
        127–9
    health education 129
    life target changing 119
    reflection 90–1
    vigilance 89
health education 121–31
    conceiving 130
    foundational 124–9

health care workers 129
    heart disease 123
    individual level 130
    indoctrination avoidance 123–4
health for all 43
    achieving 133–4
health projects, funding 78
health promotion 69, 74, 121–2
    literacy 131
    political action 130–1
    purpose 127–9
    reasoning ability 131
health services 65
    dependence on 127
    function beyond medical scope 66
    funding 130
    public/private 130
health supply 56
health systems planning 101
health visitors 127–9
    confidence 128–9
    need for coherent model 128
Healthy Cities programme 78
healthy person 7–13
healthy state 74
heart disease 54, 55
    causes 124
    health education 123
herd instinct 26, 27
Herlich, Claudine 50
HIV infection 68
housing 70, 72, 129
human bodies, medical perspective 56
human condition
    poverty 125–6
    see also potential, human
human desires 6
human dignity 62
human diversity 63
humanism 47–53, 61–3
    health increase approach 40
hygiene, improved 51

iatrogenesis 58, 59, 60
ideal state theory of health 39, 40, 41–5, 52
    conceptions of health 74–9
    implications 44
idealists, health definition 11, 12
ideology, single-minded 17
Idols, Bacon's doctrine 25–6
ignorance 105
Illich, Ivan 51, 58–61
illness 37–41
    causes 66
    chronic 54, 55
    experience as quality 39
    obstacle removal 130
    patterns 54
    prevention 119, 121
    recurrent 54, 55
immunisation campaigns 123
individuals
    community 85–6, 98–9

individuals (*cont.*)
   complexity 85–6
   health assessment 120
   health education 130
   work for health 88
inequality of opportunity 120
infection control 51–2
infectious diseases 51–2
influences on health 86–8
   bad 86–7
information 85
injury 87
inner strength 49, 50
inquisitiveness 18
instincts 57
intellectual liberation 127
intellectual stagnation 26

judgement 33–4
justice, definition 18

keywords 27–8
   see also democracy; meaning; rationality
King, Lester 38
knowledge
   institutions shaping life 130
   medical 56
   self-development 127
Koestler, Arthur 32–3

L-DOPA 48, 50
lay concepts of health 50
liabilities 120
   human potential 105
   ignorance 105
   measurement 91
life target changing 119
lifestyle 87
   affluent 11, 12, 117–18, *119*
literacy 131
living conditions 66
lost health 46
low incomes 70, 72

Mansfield, Katherine 51, 64–5
Maori activist 10, 12, 13
   work for health 116–17
Maori understanding of health 69–70, *71*, 72–3
market economy 55
materialism 46
meaning
   historical tradition 29, 34
   keywords 27–8
   legitimate 29, 82, 89
   limits 84
   philosophy in clarification 29–34
   potential 103–6
   problem of 23–36
   shifts with time 36, 66
   variety 29
measurement of health 83
medical industry 55, 56

medical interventions, harmful 58, 59, 60
medical knowledge 56
medical products 56
medical science
   approach to health increase 40, 55–8
   criticisms 56–8
   health quantification 57
   objectivity 57
   species-typical theory of health 67
medicine
   assumptions 55
   creation of health 134
   engineering 56
   health care 36
   Illich's criticisms 58–61
   magic bullets 43
   romantic science 46
   sociology 57–8
   subordination to 58
mental defect absence 25
mental disease 52
mental health 78–9
mental illness 78–9
mental well-being 42–3, 69, *71*
meta-ethics 16
metaphysical issues 16, 47
metaphysical strength 48–50, 52
Mexican peasants 50
Mill, John Stuart 107, 128, 130
Miller F. N. 38
mind concept 32
Mitchell, Jeanette 54, 55
moral rules 16
morality
   choice 131
   humanism 62

needs, basic 85
Nordenfelt, Lennart 68, 74
normality, biological 25
norms, establishment 57–8

obsessions 49
occupations 45, 66
Oliver, Michael 124
opportunity, inequality 120
optimum capacity for health 44
optimum states 66
over-industrialisation of society 59

pain
   feelings 39
   relief 60
paraplegic 8–9, 11, 12, 13
   work for health 113, *114*
Parisians, middle-class 50
Parkinsonian effects 48, 49
Parsons, Talcott 44
paternalism 127
Peery T. M. 38
personal fulfilment 46
personal goals, humanist 62
personal relationships 87

personal strength/ability 40, 41
  conceptions of health 79–80
philosophers
  changing 17
  children as 17–18
philosophy 15–21
  childhood rebellion 20–1
  clarification 16–17, 20
  clarification of meaning 29–34
  end-product 17
  exercising abilities 19
  as form of thinking 20
  of health ix
  nature of health 15–16
  need for 19–21
  power of 16
  professional 19, 20
  questions 18
  student of 19
  thinking 35
physical defect absence 25
physical well-being 42, 69–70, 71
planning, participatory 102
Plato 18
points of reference, shared 29
Polanyi, Michael 30
Polemachus 18
political action 130
political ideals 131
pollution 52, 66
Popper, Karl 30
potential 106
  meaning 103–6
potential, human 43, 64, 103–7
  achievement 64, 105, 106
  assessment 104–5
  assumptions 103–4
  awareness of community 99
  choice 107
  ethics 107
  fulfilling 95
  group 96
  health education/promotion 129
  health worker role in achievement
    106
  indefinite number 104
  latent 43
  liabilities 105
  measurement 104
  negative 105
  obstacle removal 64
  paraplegic case study 113
  positive 105
  realising 125
  realistic 103
  species-typical 106
  see also biological potential
power to achieve/to truly be 65
privilege, obtaining 6
propaganda 123–4
psychiatry 78–9
public health 56

quality of life 131, 134
  measurement 92
  state of health 65, 119
questioning, philosophical 18
questions, children's 17–18

rational person 28
rationality 28
realism, human potential 103
reasoning ability 131
received wisdom acceptance 26
recollections, mythical 43
reflection
  health care workers 90–1
  work for health 134
reserves of health 50
resource allocation
  participatory planning 101
  political 130
rights of individuals 74
roundness 83–4

Sacks, Oliver 46, 48–50, 52, 125
sanitation, improved 51
scientific method 52
self-care 60, 61, 127
self-determination 62
self-development 125, 126
  ability 25
  benefits 127
  latent ability 62
  reduced dependence on health services
    127
self-education 17
sick role 44, 45
sleeping sickness 48–50
smokescreens 27
smoking 87
social change 93–4
social class 54, 55, 87
  differences 53–4
social conditions 72
social duties, excused from 44
social research 54
social role, functioning in 11, 12
social science
  achieving health 55
  health definition 11, 12
social well-being 42
society
  over-industrialisation 59
  suppression of philosophy 17
sociology
  health increase approach 40, 53–5
  medicine 57–8
Socrates 18
  analogues of squares 89–91
  roundness 83–4
Solzhenitsyn, Alexander 26–7
species-typical theory of health 67–8
  incorporation into foundations theory
    106
spirit, human 48

spiritual being 57
spiritual strength 48, 49, 50
spiritual wellbeing 69, *71*
state of health 65
    assessment 91–4, 96–7
        measure 91–2, *93*
    case studies 110–19
    measurement 109
    optimum 95
    variables 109
strength 81, 114
    elements 53
    inner 49, 50
    metaphysical 48–50, 52
    reserves 50, 52
    spiritual 48, 49, 50
stress 66, 87
stroke, foundations theory application
    99–102
sympathy engendering 6
syndrome 37
synthesis 32

Tengland, Per-Anders 68
theories of health xii, 37
    ability to adapt 51–2
    Caroline Whitbeck's 73–4
    commodity 39, 40, 41, 45–7, 79
    components 82–3
    disagreement acknowledgement 82
    fitness necessary to perform normal tasks
        39, 40, 41, 44–5, 79
    ideal state 39, 40, 41–4, 52, 74–9
    personal strength/ability 40, 41, 47–53,
        79–80
    realism 83
    species-typical 67–8, 106
    usefulness 83
    vital goals 68–9
    see also foundations theory of health
theorising 32, 33
theory
    articulated 31
    concept relationship 35
    formation 33
    meaning 29, 30, 35
    possession 33–4
    precursor 35
Theory of Forms 84
thinking/thought
    clarity 25
    focus 25
    philosophical 19, 20, 35
tics 49
tolerance 62
training 122
tribal memories 43

understanding
    barriers against 25, 27

lay 51
    reasoned 30
unemployment 10, 70, 72
    work for health 115–16
universal standards 58

vascular disease 52
vigilance, health care professionals 89
vital goals theory of health 68–9
vitalism 46

way of life, healthy 52
weakness 50
Werbeniuk, Bill 124
Western liberal tradition 107
Western understanding, influence on Maori
    thought 70, 72
Whitbeck, Caroline, theory of health 73–4
White, William 38
whole, meaning 24
wholeness
    concept 66
    health relationship 36
Williams, Raymond 27–8, 34
Williams, Rory 50–1
Wittgenstein, Ludwig 16–17, 20
words
    barriers against understanding 25, 27
    current usage 29
    meaning 29
work avoidance 6
work for health 4, 82
    affluent lifestyle 117–18, *119*
    cancer patient 114, *115*
    concerns 89–91
    delusions case study 110, *111*
    depression 115–16
    domestic violence 117–18, *119*
    drug dealing 116–17
    enabling 84, 92, 107
    extent 133
    goals 94
    individuals 88
    liberating 133, 134
    limits 88–91, *92*
    Maori activist 116–17
    potentials 105
    primary targets 89
    re-focusing 4
    reflection 134
    self-limiting 107
    targets 89–91
    thought 134
    unemployment 115–16
World Health Organisation (WHO)
    definition of health 41–3, 54
    mental health 78–9
    website health topics 74–8

Index compiled by Jill Halliday

9 780471 490111